*"This is a must-read book for everyone before midlife. I found a thread all the way through that kept me saying, 'Been there, done that.' I'm certain everyone else will find the same thing and can then follow it into their retirement and aging years. It will fit you whether or not you are a housewife, executive, small businessperson, union worker, teacher or whatever. There is excellent advice in this book and it is not too early to apply it to yourself, however it fits."*

—WILTON JACKSON

*"This book presents very interesting personal experience accounts of the challenges and joys of aging. It could be considered a handbook for aging gracefully."*

—SR. KATHLEEN STUPFEL, SNJM

*"Greg leaves us with a rich bibliography and practical resources to navigate the 'Golden Years.'"*

—MARY BARTHOLOMEW

*"This book tells you the benefits of keeping your glass half full instead of half empty while going through the aging process. It offers many helpful suggestions."*

—BOB HENRY

*"I found the information in the book to be helpful and accurate. I wish I had this before making our decision about retirement living."*

—VIC CHRISTIANSEN

*"Anyone who is nervous about moving into a retirement community should read this book. The positives are overwhelming."*

—DALLAS COLE

*"The book does a very good job in dealing with the various factors affecting a decision to move to community living. For many, giving up their houses is very hard but they're relieving their children of a large burden later on. My kids have frequently thanked me for saving them from that distasteful task."*

—JEANNE WOLF

*"This book is great! It would have been a great help to me 30-40 years ago. I would have been able to use the wonderful advice it provides. I'll make sure my children read it."*

—HILDA KULLBERG

*"The author has a lively style of presentation that makes a potentially dull subject interesting and easy to read. Anyone planning on living to or beyond retirement will profit from the author's insights."*

—STEVE KORSAK

*"This will be a great book to give to your children or friends who may be considering a move into a continuing care retirement community."*

—MARGERY BOYDEN

*"This is a must read book. It is a page turner, interesting, informative and well researched. When you finish it you will want to read it again."*

—LILLIAN COPPOCK

*"This book represents an open-minded review of the transition everyone has to face."*

—ISHBEL MURRAY

*"This book by Greg Hadley is for those seeking a cultural, spiritual, social, physical and educational review in their later years. Autumn comes; leaves fall."*

—MARGARET DILLON

*"Greg Hadley's book gives a blueprint for gracious living to those who are approaching old age. It is a must-read for anyone contemplating retirement."*

—JUNE MCALLISTER

*"In this book, Greg Hadley has given us an insider's true evaluation and appreciation for the trials and rewards of retirement and especially the necessity for planning and foresight for those 'golden years.'"*

—VIRGINIA CAMPBELL

# Aging:
## The Autumn Phase of Life

by

GREG HADLEY

*To Sr. Barbara —*
*Celebrate Life !*
*Greg Hadley*

Hadley, Greg [1934 –    ]
Aging: The Autumn Phase of Life / Greg Hadley—1st edition

ISBN: 1-4505-7432-7

Printed in the United States of America
First edition

# OTHER BOOKS BY GREG HADLEY

*Fundamentals of Baseball Umpiring*
(In the National Baseball Hall of Fame, Cooperstown, New York)

*Common Problems; Common Sense Solutions*
(Translated into Chinese for distribution and sale in Asia-Pacific region)

*100 Everyday Epiphanies:*
    *Simple Events That Can Inspire Prayer*

*God's Words to My Heart*

# TABLE OF CONTENTS

# FOREWORD

For the past twenty-five years, I have been actively engaged in the retirement and senior health care fields. It has been my life and my passion as well as my profession, and currently, I am the executive director of Mary's Woods at Marylhurst, a continuing care retirement community in Lake Oswego, Oregon. In my work, I have watched the aging and aged population face a variety of challenges as they enter the later phases of life. I have worked with these people closely and understand that the issues to be dealt with extend beyond physical health. Questions related to psychological, emotional, attitudinal and spiritual well-being can be equally complex and intricate.

I can also tell many stories about people who have failed to deal with these issues at the appropriate time. In many cases, their situations did not turn out so well for them, their loved ones, their extended families, or those providing care.

I began reading this book to gain insights, which I hoped to share with the people I serve. I soon realized that I was seeing something much more than I had expected. Greg has done a masterful job at walking the reader through the journey of life. As someone well into this journey (I'm fifty-four years old and just became a grandfather!) it felt like staring into a mirror of my own life. Greg comprehensively outlines the truth about aging, covering not only our inevitable physical decline but also examining its other equally important aspects. His analysis supports the advice we generally fail to heed until these inevitable realities are upon us.

If you embrace the essence of this book, you will find yourself much better prepared for the road ahead. You will be equipped to approach the autumn phase of life stronger emotionally, spiritually, financially, and yes, even physically. Greg goes beyond merely sharing experiences. He reaches further to extract practical lessons learned along his own personal journey. He offers words of wisdom and suggestions that make us ponder aging in a new light; even with my extensive professional experience in this field, Greg opened my eyes to things I had never really paid attention to in the past. He puts the reality of aging into new perspective and shows how each of us can embrace this phase of our lives.

I especially appreciated the chapter devoted to financial considerations. In the very tough economic times of 2008 and 2009, I have watched the painful strain placed on seniors as they attempt to manage their resources. Greg's straightforward and easy-to-understand advice will be helpful. While money does not make us happy, it is an important part of how we will happily spend our latter years.

In short, *Aging: The Autumn Phase of Life* is full of wisdom, knowledge, and poignant stories. This book is a must-read for everyone approaching the latter stages of their lives, or who have parents currently facing the challenges that older folks must deal with. Greg's book will make the journey much easier, as it offers helpful information, useful strategies, and profound insights. And above all, it enriches the readers with a sense of security and peace while dealing with this phase of our human journey.

*Edward Mawe, M.Ed., N.H.A.*
Executive Director, Mary's Woods at Marylhurst,
Lake Oswego, Oregon

# PREFACE

*"Getting old I can handle. Being old is the problem."*
—Rabbi Albert Lewis

Aging, both in concept and reality, is the subject of many clichés. Among the most often-used is, "It sure beats the alternative." You picked up this little book for one of several reasons. You may be part of the general population who has reached "old age"—whatever that means. Or, you may not be there yet but wondering about the aging process. As Father John LaFarge, S. J. says in his book, *Reflections on Growing Old*, you may be interested in the question of old age for the simple reason that one of these days you, too, are going to get there. Perhaps you have aged parents and you're trying to understand how to deal with the effects of aging on their lives—and yours. You might find yourself on the cusp of the "aging phase" and want to see what it may hold for you.

What you will find here is my personal story about aging and the stories of my friends and neighbors. Joan Chittister, in her wonderful book, *The Gift of Years: Growing Old Gracefully,* says that there are three stages of "old" in our society: the *young-old*, sixty-five to seventy-four years old; the *old-old*, seventy-five to eighty-four;

and the *oldest-old*, age eighty-five and over. Statistically, I am about halfway through the process at age seventy-five. However, I stipulate that only God knows how much further I will proceed in this phase of my human experience. If I am granted more years of life, I have absolutely no idea what challenges I may face—medically, financially, emotionally, spiritually, or psychologically. I do have many strong opinions about how to deal with certain aspects of aging; I will share them with you to provide a point of view for your consideration.

This is not a book about gerontology, geriatrics, or health sciences for the aged. Nor will you find much statistical or anthropological data about the aging process. I believe the most important parts of this book are the personal stories, so I will discuss how physical aging has affected my friends, my wife, and me, and how it might affect you. I am not a trained psychologist or social scientist, but I hold convictions about the emotional, spiritual, attitudinal, and psychological components of aging that I will develop. As Father LaFarge states, "Age both robs us and enriches us." I have found this to be true on many levels. For instance, I may offer no advice about specific investment strategies, but will discuss important financial considerations.

I find autumn to be the most pleasant and refreshing of our seasons. The crisp, sunlit days, the cool nights, beautiful colors on the deciduous trees, walking through the crunch of fallen leaves and wonderful aromas—all contribute to autumn's appeal. We experience a new phase of our life as we reach our advanced years. These autumn years can be very affirming, pleasant and fulfilling, a capstone to a well-led life. Unfortunately, they may become an anguished period of doubts, anxieties and suffering. Which road we take is only partially in our control. We can, however, pull many levers that help direct our path through aging. In other words, I am convinced a proactive approach is better than a passive one. While there are many events I cannot influence, there are some things I can affect.

Everyone gets old, physically, if they live long enough. Current actuarial tables set the life span for females at about 80 years old, and 77 for men. Due to medical advances, improved nutrition and awareness of what a healthy lifestyle entails, we now often hear of people living to 100 years and more. It is likely that life span will further increase in the future. However, we must accept the fact that none of us gets out of here alive.

As we approach the end of earthly life, we can choose to curl up in the fetal position and await our ultimate fate. Or, we can decide to live these final years, months, and days as productively and pleasantly as possible, all the while building our legacy for future generations to emulate and admire. Most would choose the latter strategy but understand this may not be their call ultimately.

It's tough to be too exuberant when you realize the endgame is the physical death of the human body. In spite of that fact, I will do my utmost to offer a positive, enthusiastic approach to each topic I address. I am not a Pollyanna, either. Aging is serious business, not just for the ones going through it but also for the family, friends, and loved ones who surround that person.

The place where I live is like a test laboratory for the

aging event. Mary's Woods at Marylhurst in Lake Oswego, Oregon is a beautiful continuing care retirement facility that houses about 350 people living independently and another 100 or so that are in assisted living, skilled nursing, or a special memory unit. The average age of those living here independently is 84. In the four years we have resided here, we have found our neighbors to be accomplished, generous, friendly, interesting, loving, and full of fascinating narratives about their lives. I thank the residents of Mary's Woods for making my life here so abundant.

Throughout this book, you will read several of the stories that my neighbors and friends have shared with me. I hope their words will paint a rich collage for you that describes various aspects of the aging process. Yes, aging beats the alternative—most of the time. As we learn when examining the aging process, there can be things worse than death to deal with. In *Reflections on Growing Old*, Father LaFarge asks:

> Why must I change so much? Why must I grow weak, why do I have to resign from occupations? Why do I find myself becoming confused, forgetting names and misaddressing envelopes?

We ask ourselves these questions while at the same time expressing our gratefulness as we pass through the aging phase of our lives. It is human nature, I guess, to cling to life and do everything possible to extend our time here on Earth. Yet I think we should add a few caveats to this wish: that we may live that extended life in relative good health; free from chronic pain, emotional suffering, and spiritual anxiety; and surrounded by people who love and cherish us. Some of us may not be so fortunate. So we need to learn to live with the hand that is dealt to us. Life—from conception to natural death—is precious. This book is about making every effort to deal with our allotted time on earth in an exemplary way. To do this well is a significant challenge.

# ACKNOWLEDGEMENTS

When we pick up a book to read, we may say, "The author must have put a lot of time and effort into getting this published." That may be true, but publication is never a one-person accomplishment. This book would not have been possible without contributions from a large number of people. Most of them are residents of Mary's Woods at Marylhurst, in Lake Oswego, Oregon. I interviewed these residents and they shared with me many stories, impressions and their views about aging. Some of the conversations were emotional, touching, personal, and candid. While we are neighbors and friends, I asked them to reveal some fairly private stuff. (You can find a full list of these questions in this book's appendix). I believe most people were quite open with me, but if anything was held back—as I'm sure must have been the case sometimes—I don't blame the interviewees. I probably would have done the same thing if the roles had been reversed.

I must express how deeply grateful I am to the following people for their time and contributions to this work: Mary Bartholomew, Margery Boyden, Virginia Campbell, Vic Christiansen, Dallas Cole, Cary and Lillian Coppock, Margaret Dillon, Sterling Dorman, Bob Henry, Tye and

Betty Lou Hutchens, Wilton Jackson, Steve Korsak, Hilda Kullberg, Philip and Dorothy Martin, June McAllister, Ishbel Murray, Edith Pattillo, Sr. Kathleen Stupfel, SNJM, Jeanne Wolf, and Dorothy Gornick (the only interviewee who does not live in Mary's Woods). I hold you all in special esteem—you are wonderful!

Having thanked these people by name, I must also tell you how indebted I am to so many other Mary's Woods residents who have shared their personal stories with me over the years. Just because I did not arrange a personal interview with everyone does not mean that my knowledge was not greatly enhanced by all the unnamed people who have helped me to understand the dynamics of aging, especially in community. I am truly blessed because of my many friends.

Thanks also to Ed Mawe, executive director of Mary's Woods, who generously wrote the foreword, and to Cheri Mussotto-Conyers, director of marketing at Mary's Woods, who provided the afterword. Their contributions are deeply appreciated. This book would not have been possible without the editing work of Sarah Cypher. As I have said before, good editors—and Sarah is terrific—keep writers like me humble as they point out errors in logic, grammar, word usage, and syntax. Sarah's work added immeasurably to the quality of this book.

As I get older, this work of writing becomes harder and more tedious. This is my fifth book. I am grateful to my wife, Evie, who is patient with me as I sit at the computer day and night struggling to get the right words into an electronic file. My being tethered to this machine has disrupted Evie's schedule more than once, I'm sure.

Thanks for being so understanding, dear Evelyn.

Finally, to all my friends and neighbors who were aware of this project and continuously encouraged me and cheered me on, many thanks are offered. I hope this effort meets everyone's expectations.

I dedicate this book to St. Anthony of Padua, patron saint of the elderly and St. Francis de Sales, patron saint of writers.

*Greg Hadley*

CHAPTER 1:

# WHEN DID I GET OLD?

*"For the unlearned, old age is winter;*
*for the learned, it is the season of the harvest."*
—THE TALMUD

Evie and I married in 1957 when I was twenty-three and she was twenty-two. We were—and looked—very young on our wedding day. Fast-forward twenty-five years: that once-young couple now had six children, many memorable life events, and boxes full of unsorted photographs, mementos, and other saved "junk." About the time of our silver anniversary, my wife declared that this memorabilia needed to be organized into a system that captured our family history, the development of the kids, the fun places we had visited, and other highlights from our first quarter-century together.

We made a fateful deal. She would begin going through these saved pictures and accumulated memorabilia from our own childhoods and continue right through our 25th anniversary while creating appropriate scrapbooks. Once that was accomplished, I would keep the scrapbooks current as the ensuing years rolled by.

I secretly thought I had gotten the better part of this arrangement. Sorting all the old pictures, getting the dates right, choosing what to save and what to throw away looked like a monumental job to me. You can also imagine the enthusiasm of a young married couple having a lot of kids; the camera always seemed to be out and both of us were quick to click off another picture of a cute infant or toddler. The material saved must have included well over two thousand photographs.

Evie waded into the task and bought the scrapbooks, and about six months later, the project began to take shape. We had agreed on one condition: No photo would be posted in the books unless we could identify all the people in it. Both of us had inherited pictures from our parents or siblings containing groups of unidentifiable friends or distant relatives. Never again, we promised each other, would a picture be catalogued without appropriate identification.

The first scrapbook started with our own early lives. Evie displayed facing pages depicting every aspect of our lives at about the same ages. This parallel presentation continued through our high school years. The account merged when we got to university and met one another. From there forward, it became one story. We proceeded through our years at university, fell in love, and planned to marry shortly after our graduation from the University of San Francisco.

Evie did a wonderful job on her part of the bargain. There was even a bonus: she set aside duplicate and extra pictures for each of our kids so that they could individually create personal books of their growing-up years. A couple of the youngest children complained that there weren't nearly as many pictures available of them as had been given to the older siblings. We confessed to a certain amount of camera fatigue on our part as more children joined our family. More kids meant fewer pictures—maybe it was something about the younger ones looking like the older ones and doing pretty much the same cute things. Boring. Anyway, Evie's efforts consumed about five scrapbooks from our own youth through our 25th anniversary, and it was fun to relive our experiences with an occasional visit to these living history binders on our shelves.

Now, it was time for me to take over. Each year thereafter, I gathered all the pictures, ticket stubs, postcards from faraway places, and other mementos into new scrapbooks. I was careful not to fall too far behind. As my kids grew, they teased me about having the current year's scrapbook completed three months in advance of the end of the year. We added yet another variable: When we took a big vacation or tour (such as to Great Britain, Ireland, Germany, Switzerland, Australia, New Zealand, Japan, Thailand, and Mexico), we would add a separate book containing a detailed log of the trip as well as photographs and other mementos.

This practice has continued to the present day. As our travels diminished and our activities slowed down, we don't have as much to chronicle as we used to. Additional camera fatigue, probably. I now get two to three years into a single scrapbook. Our collection currently numbers almost thirty books. When we sold our home in 2005 and moved to this retirement community, lots of downsizing was required. We made a deal with our local daughter, Leigh Anne. She could keep one of our nice bookcases that we otherwise planned to sell, if she would provide a home for all our scrapbooks. It's a good arrangement. Often, when visiting her, we go to the upstairs room where the books are housed. It is a pleasure to look back on specific times and recall all the things that happened. Some of the color in the old photos is fading, however. Evie and I find that, in many respects, we are fading, too—in real life.

Why am I telling you all of this about our family scrapbooks? Looking at these old books and then glancing into a mirror each morning is a perfect allegory for the title of this chapter, "When Did I Get Old?" I can track my physical growth from a young boy of three or four years old through the teenage years, on to young adulthood, early middle age, fifties and sixties and finally to my current age of seventy-five.

Of course, the pictures document the physical changes that have occurred, but they are one-dimensional because they only show differences in body shape and size, coloring of hair, and gravity's effects on sagging chins, stomachs, and cheeks. Pictures do not record the emotional, spiritual, psychological, and attitudinal changes which also have taken place. So, even though I study these old books we created, they do not help me answer the question posed in this chapter.

* * *

I was curious what my neighbors and friends thought; had they pondered this concept of getting old? So, the first query I made in my interviews was, "When did you realize you had gotten old?" I received some interesting comments. Ishbel ("Call me Ish") Murray possesses an athletic posture that belies her ninety years. "I don't think of myself as old even now," she said. "I've really enjoyed 'the trip' and have done everything I was supposed to do, I believe. I feel my work is complete, but God apparently wants me to stick around a while—I don't know why."

June McAllister is a perfect model for everyone's grandma: short, slightly stooped, with a big, friendly smile for all, and inquisitive eyes. "I found out I was old about five years ago when I got a case of shingles. That was just terrible! When that happened, I knew age had caught up to me. The other signs have all been gradual; I just can't do as much as I used to. Having said that, I still don't really *feel* old, although my body keeps telling me otherwise. But, as each new day comes, I say to myself— everything is OK and 'I'm just me.'"

Steve Korsak is one of the younger Mary's Woods residents. Trim, handsome, and athletic, Steve has lived with Parkinson's disease for seventeen years. The malady has slightly limited his speech and he has a hitch to his gait. Formerly a professional ski racer and racecar driver, Steve says old age "was not something I discovered; it was imposed on me," when his illness was diagnosed. Even so, he is active and almost frenetic with his daily exercise regimen. Steve claims to live by the three following mantras: "Time is not money; time is *time*;" "You only live once;" "You don't get to come back." He says, "I've had fourteen very good years since being diagnosed. The last three have presented me with more difficulties, but I'm still doing my best."

Wilton Jackson is a resident in his late eighties, and is very fit and trim—he looks more like a seventy-year-old. He speaks with a slight Western drawl. He states that he discovered old age at eighty-four while panning for gold in an Idaho stream. Picking up a rock that contained flecks of the precious metal, he tried to take a whack with his pick—and found he couldn't do it anymore. "I had to admit it—my body had gotten old," said Wilton.

Virginia Campbell, a remarkably sharp-witted ninety-nine-year-old, responded emphatically, "No! No! I am *not* old; I may be decrepit but I am not old." Virginia's speech is clear and firm, and the stories she relates are filled with memories of her past accomplishments and those of her recently deceased spouse, Herald. Yes, Virginia admits, there are all kinds of physical signs that she has lived ninety-nine years. In spite of this long list of "annoyances," as Virginia describes them, she claims her memory is as good, or better, than it once was and she still finds interest and challenge in a whole raft of activities. You will hear more about Virginia later in this book.

Bob Henry, a big man with a booming, raspy voice and an ever-present smile, said old age approached gradually, but golf sealed the deal. "We play a weekly game in the summer and fall on a local nine-hole course and I must ride a cart to make it around. That told me I had gotten old. But, other than that, I still enjoy life and I don't really feel old."

Joan Chittister, in *The Gift of Years*, summarizes this idea perfectly:

[Those] who do not feel old, whatever their chronological age, one day realize with a kind of numbing astonishment that they have not managed to elude it. They are older than they ever thought they could possibly become. They are now called "seniors" or "the elders" or "the older generation," even "elderly," by the young ones around them, despite the fact that inside themselves they feel no different now than they did a year ago. Except for the telling of the years, of course. And, in the end, those make all the difference.

*     *     *

Besides the hazy threshold of old age, what also interests me are the lessons to be learned from our memories—when we draw on events we recall with complete clarity. "Just like yesterday," as the saying goes.

I can recall situations from first grade when I was probably six years old. My teacher, a young nun at St. Thomas the Apostle Grade School in Minneapolis, called my mother in for a conference. It seems that I had been both careless and delinquent in cutting out and pasting my lessons into a workbook. I can clearly recall where I was seated at the nun's desk relative to my mother and the teacher. Sister explained my poor performance in exquisite detail to my mother. The humiliation I felt was vivid, being singled out for my lazy work habits and failure to keep up with the rest of the class on assignments. What I am relaying here is not fuzzy or vague; it is crystal clear in my mind's eye almost seventy years later. I learned a lesson that afternoon which stuck with me the rest of my life: Only my best effort would be acceptable in any future endeavor. I did not like the criticism I received and I never wanted my mother to be ashamed of me in the future.

This is not the only incident that is vividly real to me. A kiss from my eighth-grade sweetheart; several baseball games where I made some memorable plays; a number of events in college; a speech made in Australia; a thunder and lightning storm in Cuernavaca, Mexico; and a fall I took in a bank parking lot. Those things, and others, are vivid to me. Don't ask me to remember a lot of detail about my wedding, the first ten years of our married life, most of my business associations or special birthdays, anniversaries, or other key events. It's not like I don't remember most of those things, but my recollection is hazy and incomplete. I have a sense that many readers can list the same type of lucid events in their own lives.

So, examining our memory banks may offer some different insights, but they offer little help in answering the question, "When did I get old?"

What about looking at my life through the prism of emotional, spiritual, psychological, and attitudinal changes that have occurred over time? I was aware of certain events that changed me. As a young father and breadwinner, I felt a lot of pressure to be successful in my role. When times were tough at work at IBM, I knew I did not have the option to fail. It seemed that each year or two brought us another child to raise. While I wasn't nearly empathetic enough with Evie's challenges at home, I often felt the weight of the world when considering the financial aspects of our married life. I can remember using my lunch hour to attend Mass in downtown San Francisco pleading with God to help me accept my responsibilities and lead me to success in my work, so that I could care for my growing family.

God must have answered my pleas. In 1963, I received my first promotion at IBM that elevated me to a management job. Instead of relying mostly on sales commissions, I was now on a handsome salary; our financial picture suddenly looked brighter. So much brighter, in fact, that Evie and I purchased an upgraded home on the San Francisco peninsula. This economic good fortune was negatively offset by virtually constant travel required in the new job. I would leave home on Sunday evening or early Monday and not return until late Friday, exhausted and utterly spent. I brought little home to Evie except a suitcase of dirty laundry to be washed and readied for the next trip. It was easy to feel sorry for myself, but I had to grudgingly admit that my work, though grueling, was stimulating and rewarding. Evie, on the other hand, was stuck at home with four little children all week with no help and no one to talk to. In hindsight, I am convinced her life was enormously more strenuous and difficult than mine.

This management job I filled was normally a three-year assignment. Through good fortune and performance, I was promoted again in one year at age thirty. This time, I was to become a marketing manager in a large Los Angeles office, in charge of ten salespeople. Again, my salary increased and I also received a bonus based on how well my subordinates performed their sales jobs. Based on 1964 dollars, Evie and I were earning more money than we had ever expected to see in our lives. We moved to a lovely home in Fullerton, California and our family continued to grow and thrive. The prior year of constant travel had taken a physical toll on me but I was still young and didn't really feel that I had "lost a step." Evie loved her home, the neighborhood environment, and her social attachments, many of which evolved from our church community. In just seven years since our marriage, we had come a long way, certainly from a material standpoint.

Soon after our move, we began to experience some profound changes in our lives. My father moved in with us when he became terminally ill, and he died soon afterwards. While I did not know my father well (he and my mother divorced when I was five but remarried when I was twenty-six) he had influenced my political thinking. Dad had been fervent about politics, like my grandfather, and always preached that nothing was more important than being actively involved in party politics. I picked up on that advice and was quite committed to political activity for most of my early adult life.

My ideas started to change when I was in my late thirties. Over the next few years, my perspective on politics evolved. While I remained active in the political scene and don't believe I abandoned my principles, I no longer possessed the same partisan passion I once had. I suppose it could be said that my thinking had progressed to a more balanced position. I learned that neither major political party is right about everything all the time.

Regarding spiritual changes, Evie and I had always been observant Roman Catholics, but in 1969 we were exposed to a weekend retreat called a Cursillo that amazingly changed our religious lives—in an extremely positive way. From a spiritual point of view, we both became more mature.

During the same time I became disillusioned with working for IBM. It was standard practice at the time to move people when they were promoted. Evie was so happy in Fullerton that I knew she would be devastated if I announced another advancement—and my superiors were already talking to me about a new position located in White Plains, New York. So, I seriously considered leaving the company. On reflection, this was a life-changing decision. Here I was, working for one of the most prestigious companies in America, performing well in my current job and probably possessing an opportunity for a career of increasing responsibility, financial rewards, and corporate influence. When I told my dying father about my decision, he begged me not to throw away this wonderful opportunity. (He had gone bankrupt in the Great Depression.) But, I did leave IBM and that action significantly changed our future. That decision was a break from my youth—psychologically, at least.

There was another riveting incident that altered my view of life forever: the assassination of President John F. Kennedy. I definitely felt older after that fateful weekend concluded; my soul had been seared to its depths.

So, when did I get old?

In my thirties, I became aware that I was changing subtly. Small but telling things were happening to my body, too. Our church put on a fundraiser fashion show featuring a couple of guys (including me) to model the latest men's clothing. I was uncomfortable in the 34-inch slacks I was given to model. Imperceptibly, I was gaining a little weight.

One evening in my early forties, I was umpiring a youth baseball tournament game. I was one of the field umpires and, when I looked up into the lights illuminating the diamond, I noticed a halo surrounding the lights; my vision was just a tad fuzzy in those circumstances. Not much later, I was driving home from work in the early darkness of a winter evening and had some difficulty reading the freeway signs at long distance. I always prided myself on my keen eyesight. Was I now going to have to resort to glasses to see well? I was lucky. It took me over forty-three years to require corrective lenses. Many people find this out much earlier, even as young children.

More time passed and I was suddenly almost fifty years old. I was still vigorous and quite healthy. There were a couple of exceptions to this: slightly high blood pressure caused me to be rated on a large life insurance policy; I also experienced an occasional heart arrhythmia—which I shrugged off as nothing to worry about. I also noticed some discomfort and swelling in the knuckles of my right hand. A visit to a specialist resulted in a predictable answer: "Mr. Hadley, you are experiencing the onset of osteoarthritis." By now, I had to admit I wasn't quite as strong as I used to be. I often asked my teenaged boys to help with heavy lifting in the yard or garage. I was losing flexibility in parts of my body. And by Friday evening, after a long week at work, I was markedly more tired than I was, say, ten years earlier.

Besides the changes in my body, undeniable mileposts along the road of aging were provided by the passage of our children from toddlers, to children, then pre-teens who graduated from grammar school, teenagers who left high school for college, and eventually entered careers and marriages of their own. Nothing I can think of offers such a stark reminder that "you're getting older" than this progressive march of your children.

It sometimes seemed like I was holding on to the hand of a life clock, riding through the full circle. But that implied that everyone ages at the same rate, and that is not true. My answer to the question, "When did I get old?" is not going to be the same for you. I have often said that I know many young ninety-five-year-old people and many old seventy-five-year-old people.

* * *

Yes, we all age at a different rate—physically, emotionally, spiritually, and attitudinally. What of my friends and neighbors? How would they answer the question, "What kind of non-physical changes have you experienced in the last fifteen or twenty years?" Many paused and were initially silent. This question gets more into the core of one's being and can't be explained with the same matter-of-factness that physical changes permit. Most of my interviewees grappled with a cogent answer.

Sister Kathleen Stupfel, SNJM, is a retired but very active nun. She is friendly, loving and positive about life as she approaches her ninetieth birthday. She told me her change from an active, full schedule in her parish ministry to retirement created an emotional reaction she had not expected.

"For about a month after I left my full-time job, all I could do was sit in my chair and look out the window," Sister Kathleen told me. "I was utterly exhausted! I also learned shortly thereafter that I could still be productive and help out a couple of days a week especially with the frail elderly. But, I no longer felt I could 'take care of the whole world.'" She also said, "I found it was necessary to make emotional adjustments to match my physically aging body."

Hilda Kullberg's e-mail address is "Hurricane Hilda" and that pretty well describes this plain-talking Mary's Woods resident. Hilda admits to some attitudinal changes as she has aged. "I have learned that it isn't always wise to speak my mind. Sometimes being too forthright can cause a problem," she said. "I do tell my adult children what I think and they seem to accept my advice for what it is. My kids have been great."

Jeanne Wolf, a sophisticated and well-read woman, is somewhat emotional about her physical health. "I'm frustrated that my body will no longer do what my mind wants it to do. Honestly, I'm not reconciled psychologically with my physically deteriorating condition. At least, as long as I can continue reading, I won't be bored. Reading is my life," she said.

Bob Henry has also been through a gut-wrenching, emotional ride for the past several years. His spouse, Jean, has suffered increasingly severe Alzheimer's disease. "I have to admit—I sometimes feel depressed seeing her suffer. The gradual loss is tough. I think my attempt to accept her condition has brought me a little closer to God." (Since my interview with Bob, his wife, Jean, has died. Her memorial service was an extraordinary celebration of her life.)

Tyra ("Tye") Hutchens and his spouse, Betty Lou, sat

for my interview together. Tye, a retired medical doctor, admitted, "I do become a little depressed sometimes because of the physical disabilities I am experiencing. But my situation has made me a bit more accepting of other people and events around me, too." Betty Lou felt that her emotional and psychological reactions "have slowed down as I must increasingly address my physical limitations."

Dorothy Martin, a tall, articulate woman, painted an interesting picture about some of the mental aspects of aging. "I think our minds are like a library. When you're younger, you don't need as many shelves for your books; as you grow older, there is an expanding need for more shelves as our knowledge base grows. No wonder we forget things sometimes—there are a lot more books for us to access now!" Dorothy also told me, "I don't multi-task like I used to; that represents a big change for me as I've gotten older."

Mary Bartholomew, an attractive, petite, high-energy lady, has a very positive view of non-physical changes as she ages. Mary told me, "Before retirement, I was so busy and stressed—I had virtually no time for myself. Now, I am very relaxed and can do so many things I have always wanted to do. This is a great time in my life. Most importantly, I now have the time to develop the spiritual side of my existence."

With arguments to the contrary, like many of my friends and neighbors, I still do not feel old. I know my body sometimes aches, I don't sleep as well, I obviously need less food to sustain life, I'm growing shorter, and ailments requiring intervention from a doctor seem to be more frequent. I can't hit a golf ball nearly as far as I could, I avoid driving at night, and a brief afternoon nap is commonly required. But my mind seems to function pretty well, even though I experience brief periods of forgetfulness. I still help some business owners, offering advice about how to operate their privately held companies. I also admit that it is quite ego-boosting to be occasionally invited to speak to a group of business people or to a religious or civic group and have your ideas welcomed and applauded. In some ways, I believe I have better discernment when confronted with alternative courses of action and can process multiple concepts about the same idea simultaneously. I grasp most of what I hear and read and still have the ability, I think, to frame cogent responses to complex issues.

I don't think that chronological age has brought me more wisdom, however. In some ways, I actually am less sure of myself than when I was younger. For example, I find it harder to "read" people. Most of us routinely wear masks to keep others from finding out who we really are. Often these contrived barriers are quite effective.

* * *

The aging process also may lead us to weigh the important choices we have made. Some decisions may have been fateful. Thinking about that, I wanted to ask my neighbors a question that might indicate if any of their choices—in hindsight—should have been different. In other words, if there was one thing in life you could do over, what would it be?

Some of the answers were lighthearted. Some were

serious. Hilda Kullberg pondered a moment and then said, "I might have married my husband sooner. In hindsight, the reasons I had for waiting a year were not valid."

Wilton Jackson was more somber. "Given the chance, I might not have moved into Mary's Woods eight years ago. I think I came a few years too early. I was still enjoying the operation of my businesses and had a wonderful home, plenty of outdoor recreation opportunities, and terrific friends. But my kids wanted my wife and me to be closer, so we came when they insisted."

Vic Christiansen is a talented stained glass craftsman who produces beautiful works of art in the Mary's Woods woodshop. Vic offered a more spiritual response. "I wish I had been a better witness for Jesus Christ," Vic said. "He is the center of my life and has blessed my spouse and me so abundantly. I also wish I had learned to be more understanding of others and broadened my own professional opportunities."

Sterling Dorman is a refined and accomplished woman. A helpmate and partner to her successful but now deceased husband, Chet, Sterling was an active civic volunteer in the areas of education, the arts, and social justice. Given a chance to re-do a part of her life, Sterling told me, "I think I would have returned to school and pursued a career of public education. While I volunteered extensively in school issues, I believe I might have been even more effective. But, really, I do not have any serious regrets."

And Cary and Lillian Coppock are a delightful and deeply devoted couple whose mutual love and respect is immediately evident. Half in jest—I think—Cary told me,

"Lillian probably shouldn't have married me but 60-plus years later it seems to have worked out OK."

* * *

If you are somewhat like me, you may have seen yourself—at least parts of you—in this chapter. The process of aging is unique to each of us; there is no "age template" that stamps us out like gingerbread old people. While I am extremely grateful that I have so far been spared, I know that many readers will already have experienced serious physical complications in their later years. Things like Parkinson's, active cancer, heart disease, rheumatoid arthritis, and Type II diabetes, among many other bodily ailments, add a level of difficulty to this phase of life's journey.

Once again, I return to the original question, "When did I get old?" In the instructive little book, *Enjoy Old Age*, authors B. F. Skinner and M. E. Vaughn write,

> The prime time to think about old age, of course, is when you are old. Old age often comes as a surprise. It creeps up and catches people unawares, often because they have deliberately not watched for it. It is not the kind of thing you can learn about from early experience, because it happens only once in a lifetime.

Father John LaFarge, S. J. also provides us with some sage advice in his interesting book, *Reflections on Growing Old*. "After all, old age has its own meaning, like other phases of human life, and the wisest thing we could do, when age crept up on us, would be to explore that meaning and adopt some general plan of action so as really to profit by it." We keep trying, but can we yet answer the question, "When did I get old?"

Probably not. The answer is so complex and, as Skinner and Vaughn write, "It creeps up and catches us unawares." And, as we've seen, we must deal with more than just physical aging. The emotional, psychological, attitudinal, and spiritual dimensions of our lives also play a part.

A neighbor, Audrey McConochie, told me a touching story about traveling back East to attend the weddings of two grandsons. While she enjoyed herself, she felt a little out of place being with a lot of people she didn't know very well. She found it very comforting, she said, to return to her retirement community home. "Here I am surrounded by like minds and like souls, friends who speak my language, share in similar activities, and who comfort me when I am sick or lonely." Audrey referred to her neighbors as "last leaves," people who still cling tenuously or stubbornly to "the old forsaken bough" described in the poem of Oliver Wendell Holmes, "The Last Leaf." Those of us who have reached old age do cling together somehow, as Audrey and Holmes report. We're just not sure when old age happened to us.

Maybe the question is really not all that important anyway. Things are what they are. Perhaps you have reached seventy, eighty—or even more. If you were featured in a local newspaper article, you can be assured of being described as an "elderly person." So, like it or not, most reading this book are old by society's definition. My children think Evie and I are rapidly progressing through their self-described aging phases: Old, Older, Wrinkly,

Creaky, and Decrepit. Just wait until you get here, too, I tell them.

The most significant question may not be *when*, but *how*. How are we going to deal with the reality of being old? There are so many issues to address. The rest of this book will attempt to determine how we cope with the challenges old age brings to each of us. Consider the haunting verses from Oliver Wendell Holmes in his poem, "The Last Leaf."

> And if I should live to be
> the last leaf upon the tree,
> In the spring
> Let them smile as I do now,
> At the old forsaken bough
> Where I cling.

As we look back along the long road of life already walked, each of us seems to be merely at a different milepost, a place not necessarily dependent upon our chronological age. Some lead, others follow; the road eventually reaches a destination while at the starting point new travelers begin their own journey. A perfect continuum is in place. You have begun to meet some of the people I see and interact with every day at Mary's Woods. Their unique stories and insights confirm my belief that we are all in this thing—aging—together. This is most comforting to me. Our journey along the road may contain pleasant stretches, but is seldom smooth, often lonely, sometimes dark. And yet daylight does come and then we look around in the morning light to glimpse all the others who are traveling with us. Their presence provides us with stamina, hope and courage for the next stage of our journey. This life phase is so much easier when it is not encountered alone. Our companions—loved ones, family, friends—are important participants in our travel, encouraging and cheering us on as we approach the final way station.

CHAPTER TWO:

# OUR DISTORTED PRISM

*"All would live long but none would be old."*
—BENJAMIN FRANKLIN

At the end of the first year I worked for IBM, right out of college, I received a booklet from the personnel department. Inside, I found a complete review of all the compensation I received during the year both direct and indirect. Among other things, I could see my gross wages including sales commissions, how much money the company paid for my health insurance, workmen's compensation, and social security. In addition, the booklet predicted what my retirement benefits would be based on a steady increase in earnings. I had to laugh out loud when I saw my projected retirement date—May 1, 1999, the beginning of the first month after I had reached 65 years of age. I was twenty-two, for heaven's sake! This was January 1957. May 1, 1999 was so far in the future that I could not comprehend the date.

Every year thereafter that I worked for IBM, I received this very informative booklet that continued to focus on my distant retirement date. To me, that 1999 date was *forever* away. I felt there were several lifetimes to live before I retired, so why worry about it now? I did appreciate that IBM thought it was important, but come on, who can possibly know what is going to happen forty-three years into the future?

Of course, you probably know what really happened. I woke up one day and found that I was nearing 50. Where had the time gone? I wondered. Having left IBM long ago to pursue entrepreneurial ventures, no one was looking out for my financial retirement anymore, except me.

Raising six children with the attendant costs, especially for education, had been challenging. While I always had been able to generate income, corresponding expenses had been high. Evie used to say to me, "If our business interests are going so well, how come we never have any cash?" Other than the equity in our home and some personal property, I determined that I had very little set aside for my retirement, which I'd scheduled to occur within the next twenty years.

I was sobered by this—and a little scared, quite frankly—so I started to plan in earnest for the financial side of the retirement equation. I had some viable options, at least. My value in our business partnership had been growing. If things continued apace, my share could possibly contribute a significant six-figure sum to my personal net worth. Our home had grown substantially in value over the years; we certainly wouldn't need a six-bedroom ranch-style home when we retired. Finally, I still had a lot of good years left and was confident that I could earn—and save—even more in the coming decade or two.

I was learning that the financial aspect of retirement is a crucial element. It is so important, that a chapter of this book is devoted to it. But what I want to explore now are those years running up to retirement. There are lots of things besides finances that must be seriously considered.

*　*　*

In my fifties, I had to admit that my work was hard, stressful, and very risky. I enjoyed what I did, but owning a small, privately held company was never a smooth road to success. I could feel burnout catching up to me, and really wanted to get into something different before I reached fifty-five. By then, all the kids would be pretty well launched and Evie and I would probably be empty-nesters. We even began talking about what the future might hold, perhaps including a move away from Southern California. There were good reasons to dismiss any thoughts of a move—wonderful neighbors, a great church community, very desirable weather—but we didn't reject the idea out-of-hand.

I also started asking myself what the word "retirement" meant, and in fact, I still ponder it. Does it imply a terminal point in one's life? Most assume it is a point when daily work ceases. I wondered if, upon retirement, I would spend my time with my feet elevated in a recliner chair watching TV? Or would retirement be more about doing interesting things I never had time for during my professional career?

I believe the most insidious part of the inexorable march to this significant event in one's life is retirement's stealth—suddenly it is upon you. We complete our education; some of us marry and begin families; career development constantly demands hard work and long hours and, before one knows it, years fly by. While an end to our working life once seemed super far away, now we can see it clearly on the horizon, and most of us have given little thought to what life might be like when our professional lives conclude. And this question regarding the effects of retirement is equally valid for those who did not work outside the home, and instead devoted their lives to raising a family, maintaining active involvement in their communities, or caring for a debilitated relative.

As we heard in the previous chapter, retirement can be full of opportunity. Mary Bartholomew *loves* it. "Now I have time for travel, to develop better relationships with family and friends, to care for my body through exercise and to work on my spiritual dimension."

Sister Kathleen didn't quite retire—she changed the direction and focus of her work. She became an expert on issues related to the global environmental problems, especially from a theological perspective. She frequently speaks to groups and advocates for greater awareness and concern regarding global warming, clean water for all the world, and similar important topics.

* * *

Let's imagine our way through a proposed retirement scenario. After all, in the final stages of our career, even as we glimpse a point in the near future when our lives may change, we still view the time ahead with a certain vagueness or lack of clarity. We begin to contemplate new questions that we have not asked before. What will my health be like? Will my financial resources permit me to stop working? Are my hobbies and interests enough to keep me stimulated and busy? What about my housing needs? Do I want to consider moving closer to family members? If I am married, what about my spouse's health and feelings about a life of retirement? Where should we live?

The more organized among us may keep some notes in a file or a binder. For most, we continue to mull over the issues as time marches on. Excluding major health problems, the bulk of our thought process is focused on our potential financial situation as we now view our professional retirement on the horizon. Unfortunately, too many of us reach some transition point in our life— let's call it retirement—when change is imposed on us but we have made no plans to accommodate the new circumstances of our personal environment.

In this scenario, I am going to make a small set of assumptions to help us consider several important ideas. Say you're approaching sixty-five years old. You have decided to "call it a career" and stop working. You have determined that savings, investments, a company pension, and social security will permit you to maintain an acceptable standard of living for you and your spouse. All of these decisions have been considered and made. One day, you receive a letter from the personnel department notifying you that in ninety days you will be eligible for retirement. You are asked to come to the department to initiate the necessary paperwork related to retirement plans, benefit programs, and other details.

The letter creates a tingle of excitement in you. "I've

really made it! I can't imagine that this day has finally come!" Even though this event has been long anticipated, you rush home to show the letter to your spouse. "Can you believe it? It's really happening!" Over a celebratory glass of wine, the two of you eagerly discuss the period immediately following your actual retirement.

The first order of business planned is a one-month auto trip to visit distant children and grandchildren. It will be great to visit family without the pressure to cut things short and return to work. Plus, by driving instead of flying, you will get to see parts of the country you have never seen before except from 35,000 feet in the air. Returning from that trip, you promise yourself some badly needed golf lessons to (you hope) improve your game. Between lessons and a few rounds of golf, you have promised your spouse to take care of a number of deferred maintenance items around the house. Yes, you're actually looking forward to tackling the fairly long "honey do" list that has been posted in the garage for some time. A delicious sense of satisfaction and well-being settles in.

Everything going forward looks rosy. There will finally be time for all those things you and your spouse have always wanted—and needed—to do. No more daily work grind with its attendant stress and pressure. No more rising early, donning a suit and tie, and putting up with a nerve-wracking commute to and from work each day. No more business travel, standing in endless lines at airport security stations. No more middle seats on totally booked flights offering no food while traveling to see some client who takes ill when you arrive and cannot meet with you. No more reporting to some person fifteen years your junior who probably advanced quickly in the company because of a MBA degree from a prestigious university.

Yes, finally *you* will be your own boss. You get to set the start and stop times for all activities. You get to wear jeans and a sweatshirt every day if you want to. You can even lie down after lunch for a short nap. You can read the morning newspaper as long as you wish and have two, maybe three, cups of coffee. Yes, it all sounds quite wonderful. On top of all this, both you and your spouse are in good health. Sure, you have the aches and pains of most sixty-five-year-olds, and your hearing and eyesight have diminished a bit, but mostly you're both in very good shape. The mortgage on your home is almost paid off, too. The month after the last payment is made will be like getting another big pay raise. Yes, life is looking very good indeed. Retirement: Bring it on!

The day arrives. You clean out your desk and attend the obligatory retirement party given by your coworkers. Several people say nice things about you. There's a cake and a token gift of a dozen premium golf balls and a useful USA atlas for all your upcoming travels. Final goodbyes are said, some with handshakes and others with small hugs. You leave the building for the last time, experiencing bittersweet feelings carrying a box of personal possessions to the car. You know in your heart that you did good, conscientious work and had a successful career. You also sense that, on some level, you will miss the satisfaction that honest work provides. You have made many friends; not interacting with them daily will leave a small hole in your spirit. Oh well, you will return once in a while to have lunch with some of them; it's not as if you won't ever see them again, is it?

From a different perspective, it will be so great to put the daily responsibilities behind you. You have just recently noticed how wearying your job has become, physically, emotionally, and psychologically. To lighten that burden would be a relief. As you travel along the roadways from work toward home, you're not really sure of your feelings. Arriving home, you find a small stack of congratulatory cards and letters from family and old friends. There is also a specially prepared favorite dinner to help celebrate the last day on the job, and long-distance phone calls afterward from your kids. You feel the tension leaving your shoulders. It dawns on you that retirement has really and truly arrived.

You begin to execute your plans. The trip to visit children takes place. Sightseeing was great, visits were wonderful, and almost everything worked out as planned. Well, not quite. The trip took a little longer than scheduled. You were surprised how tired you were after just 300 miles a day of driving. Each morning you seemed to start a little later and quit a little earlier in the afternoon. It didn't make any real difference, you thought; "I'm retired and can come and go as I please." Still, the persistent fatigue surprised you.

Arriving home, you signed up for the promised golf lessons. "I can't believe how rusty my game is and how much flexibility I've lost," you mention to your spouse. Now that you're playing during the week while your weekend golf buddies are still working means that you must find some different partners for your rounds. No problem; it's good to make new friends. But, somehow it isn't the same as playing with the old gang who knew one another so well.

One can't play golf every day, so the list of home repairs and refurbishments starts to get some of your attention. The list seems longer than you had thought. While you whip through the first items, some projects turn out to be complicated. Necessary planning and several trips to the big-box home improvement store are now routine for most jobs. Everything seems to take longer than anticipated and your enthusiasm for all this work is starting to wane.

Between golf, projects at home, trips to the physical therapist (you pulled a muscle in your back on the golf driving range), and just the daily chores of living, time is flying by. "How did I ever find time for a haircut or an oil change on the car when I was working?" you muse. A friend tells you jokingly that "a train picks up speed when it's over the hill and coming down the back side." That seems to describe your life perfectly. Soon everything settles into a rhythm. Pages on the calendar turn rapidly. You are now living in the autumn of your life.

If you are already retired, I hope you found parts of the preceding little story that resonated with your own experiences. If you are still anticipating your retirement date, it may give you a small hint about what may lay ahead. I raise these issues because they represent a preface to some significant changes that are occurring in your life. One of the most profound truisms about aging is this: *Nothing stays the same.*

And therein lies the greatest challenge that many older folks must deal with as time goes on. The ancient

Hebrew saying, "This, too, shall pass," expresses the idea equally well. As we will see, these concepts become crucial in developing our life strategy. And yet, we will also note that our failure to recognize their meanings can cause devastating results for us during the final stages of our lives.

* * *

Here is the second chapter of our little hypothetical story about life after retirement. It is now ten years later. Many things have happened to our hypothetical couple since that fateful day when retirement living began. There has been lots of interesting and fun travel. Visits to foreign countries, several relaxing cruises, more opportunities to be with children and grandchildren— and all have been enjoyable.

Other good things have occurred, too. Golf and home repairs have been supplemented by a deep involvement in volunteering at local hospitals and homeless shelters. You and your spouse now spend a substantial amount of time helping out in worthwhile civic programs. You're proud of the fact that your efforts assist others who may not be as fortunate as you are.

There have been some less than positive events, too. Your spouse underwent hip replacement surgery to substitute a piece of titanium for the original equipment. Rehab was very long and torturous, and some stiffness and pain still linger. You were diagnosed with prostate cancer. Fortunately, the doctors caught it early and a radical prostatectomy removed all traces of the tumor. However, there are still some issues related to bladder and bowel incontinence and sexual function. Both of you have noticed the onset and discomfort of osteoarthritis, and your eye doctor is monitoring cataracts that both of you are developing.

Comparing today to that magic day of retirement some years back, you are both doing pretty well, but there are distinct signs that your physical condition is slipping. Again, you find it easy to rationalize this situation by saying, "Compared to many of our friends, we seem to be doing very well—" and now comes the crucial modifier— "and we expect it will stay that way into the future."

That last phrase gets most people into a lot of trouble. I contend nothing is so detrimental to successfully navigating old age than the idea that you are somehow exempt from aging and the attendant changes it demands of your lifestyle. Denial can get any of us into trouble. Why? Because the assumption is incorrect! Each new day brings changes, some that are imperceptible, but changes nonetheless. Our misguided thinking can cause us to ignore the "what's next" part of our life.

Here's the mistaken line of thinking. If things are going to be pretty much the same, why should I think about or plan too far ahead? Therefore, I won't worry about the future state of my health; my potential need for some level of care as times goes on, the possibility of downsizing while I still have the energy to do it, or making different living arrangements that will better reflect my future needs. It's just easier to say, "I'm feeling OK, life continues to be pretty good, I can still get around and I enjoy my nearby friends, family, an occasional trip, and the comfort of my home and possessions. Why should I borrow trouble by trying to change any of that?"

As C. Northcoat Parkinson wrote, "delay is the deadliest form of denial." When we delay planning for the future we engage in potentially risky behavior. I can speak with firsthand knowledge about the devastating effects of this mindset. One of our daughters was forced by circumstances to arrange increasingly more urgent levels of care for her mother-in-law, who suddenly became very ill. Within 120 days, this elderly woman went from generally acceptable functioning to near-death.

All the warning signs had been present well before the onset of trouble. Observable confusion, the possibility of early dementia, and decreasing concern for her personal hygiene should have set off alarms within the family. While there was some worrying, there was also inertia. Things weren't going well but there hardly seemed to be an emergency situation, either. That was true—until the emergency hit. From that point forward, all family energy and resources were devoted to seeking and arranging the appropriate levels of care as the situation swiftly deteriorated.

It is impossible to adequately describe the level of physical, emotional, and financial exhaustion this situation caused. Could it have been avoided? Probably. If the mother-in-law had been directed to a different type of care center as soon as her condition became noticeable (she was living in an independent living facility when all this happened), some of the trauma might have been mitigated. But that is moot, since no advance action was taken. Who knows how it would have turned out in the end? The point is: to delay dealing with an upcoming problem is a terrible form of denial.

Case number two. My brother and his wife lived in a Rocky Mountain city. He was ten years older than I. Through a relative, I was informed that he had been observed driving somewhat dangerously and erratically. I was urged to visit my brother and see for myself what was going on. When my wife and I did so, we were concerned with what we found. Their three-story home of forty-plus years, with its steep stairs, had become a hazard. The house had four bedrooms and a large yard to maintain. Now in his eighties, this was becoming too much for my brother and his wife to handle.

We also noticed a deficit in their nutrition; both my brother and his wife were extremely thin and suffering from medical issues, some of which were severe. We gently urged them to consider selling their home and moving to a retirement community, where proper levels of care would be available for them as they aged. We had even arranged tours of nearby facilities that might be suitable for them after they left their home.

My sister-in-law was particularly resistant. She said there was no way that they could downsize from their current home. When pressed, she admitted that most of their "stuff" was pictures, mementos, etc., that had been accumulated over their fifty-plus years of marriage. Exasperated and quickly losing my patience, I asked whether or not their two children were aware of this "stuff" and whether or not they wished to inherit the items after the parents passed on. The answer was no. I rather insensitively suggested that it would become a question of who would fill up the dumpster, the parents or the children. As you can imagine, this careless statement did not improve my argument. Further, I suggested that a continued denial was foolhardy. I stated—again indelicately—that time was their enemy. This was the final indignity to my sister-in-law.

"Who are you to tell me how much time I have left?" she blurted out. Needless to say, nothing came of our visit except very hurt feelings, the result of my lack of empathy and poor choice of words.

This situation ended badly, too. Finally, after their children intervened, my brother and his wife moved into a retirement community two years later, but only when the situation deteriorated further. My sister-in-law survived only a few months, succumbing to a massive stroke. Soon thereafter, the care center notified the children that my brother's condition had so declined that he could no longer stay there. The kids undertook a mission similar to my daughter's, and after some very difficult searching, eventually found a place for my brother. He, too, survived for only a short period of time. Had my advice been more effective and more sensitive, my dear brother and his wife might have enjoyed at least a couple more years together without the stresses of housekeeping and independent self-care.

Case number three. When my wife and I decided to move to a continuing care retirement community in our early seventies, most of our friends (also in their seventies) and some of our family looked at us askance. "Why in the world would you make such a move? You're still young, have your health, live in a beautiful home and remain active—and you want to move to such a place?"

I do not want to sound self-righteous here. Our decision to sell our home, downsize, and move to a retirement place was right for us. It might not be right for others, either now or in the future. Also, what we chose to do was just one of many alternative courses of action—some of which I discuss in the next chapter.

What did surprise us, however, was our friends' reaction. When we asked them what they had planned for their future, we pretty much got blank stares. It appeared to us that many had accepted that false assumption: "Things are OK now and we don't see any significant change happening in the foreseeable future." We heard a lot of comments like: "Maybe we'll consider something like you have done in five or ten years." "There's no way we would be willing to downsize now." "If something happened to us, our children would take care of us." "You live in a place where death is around every corner."

At this writing, we have lived in our retirement community for about four years. Some of our friends who scoffed at our decision have gone through serious medical episodes. Others have experienced the loss of a spouse. We don't offer these examples to justify our choice. We merely point out that, in the final analysis, *we are not in control of events.* In my opinion, planning for "what's next" is just a prudent thing to do.

*   *   *

Our friends living in Mary's Woods revealed their own reasons for moving here. Essentially, everyone I interviewed was asked, "Given all the alternatives, why did you decide to come to a place like Mary's Woods? Was there one overriding reason for your decision? How much did your family influence your decision process?"

A lovely woman resident who is articulate and talented told me, "I knew I needed to leave my home and find a retirement community to move to. But everyplace I visited left me feeling depressed—until I walked into Mary's Woods. There was just something—a spirit, I think—that totally charmed me. I fell in love with the place right away. I'm not a Catholic, but I just knew this is where I was supposed to be."

Philip Martin, a tall, angular retired Presbyterian minister, knew about retirement communities because of relatives who had lived in them. "One thing was quite important to us—we wanted to find a non-profit operation. We also liked this community [Lake Oswego, Oregon]. While our children did not influence our decision, we did feel that we had done them a great favor by settling into a continuing care retirement community that could care for us through the end of our days. I must tell you, however, as a Presbyterian minister, I never thought I would retire to a place that once served as a Catholic convent!"

Bob Henry's personal experience influenced his decision, too. He watched his parents refuse to leave their family home at a time when they needed help with daily living. "It turned out that my folks needed full-time help for over their last three years. That whole time was traumatic for my siblings and me. I knew I would never put my kids through something like that," Bob said. "To me, that made our decision to move to Mary's Woods easy."

Wilton Jackson told me that his children handled virtually all the moving arrangements. There was some discussion regarding the costs associated with such a move. Wilton rightly observed that conversations about money among family members can sometimes be problematic. Wilton reminded me that "the most tender part of the human body is the one that connects the heart to the pocketbook."

These neighbors made informed and carefully thought-out decisions. But, we do know that it is easy to view the future and make choices by looking through a distorted prism. Not one of us knows what the future holds. Evie and I have always considered this fact to be a great blessing. But as we approach advanced age, we can make a serious mistake by burying our heads in the sand, denying that changes are happening to us or that we are truly in control of future events. There is an old saying: "If you want to give God a good chuckle, tell Him what your plans for the future are."

Give thought to your future personal strategy. Consider all the options for living a happy, healthy life while advancing in years. Try to avoid being overtaken by events that will limit your options. The objective is to live this autumn phase of life well, productively, and with grace. What is your plan to achieve that goal?

# CHAPTER 3:

## EXAMINING ALTERNATIVES

*"To me, old age is always fifteen years older than I am."*
——Bernard Baruch
(also Oliver Wendell Holmes in a slightly different form)

The very first step in your "what's-next" planning is to come to grips with the fact that time and events move on inexorably. *Almost* everyone accepts this fact, eventually. Unfortunately, some remain in denial and others wake up to their circumstances when it is often too late to do much about it.

Evie and I started to think about these issues seriously in our late sixties and early seventies. We lived in a wonderful single-story home and could have continued staying there for a long time. We had begun the process of hiring people to help us with chores that we used to take care of personally. Gardeners, arborists, and trades-people visited frequently, and their help made our lives much easier—although more expensive. But, we also understood that we couldn't stay in our home forever.

Issues related to mobility, health care, or extended personal service requirements were almost certain to increase in the future, like it or not. Both of us had already experienced multiple surgeries and our general health profiles contained some issues that were probably not going to get a lot better over time. Expecting our one local daughter, Leigh Anne, to provide some or all of these care services to us was not an alternative for us. So, we began to examine the range of options available while looking at the pros and cons of each.

In order to make this discussion more generic (and not just about our personal decision) I again use the example of a hypothetical aging couple ensconced in their home of many years. It has become apparent to them that the house is too big for their needs, yard and garden maintenance becomes more difficult every year, and many repairs are no longer "do it yourself" projects but require outside contractors or family members to complete. In addition, old time neighbors are dying or moving away, regular service providers like doctors and dentists are retiring, as well as church pastors. So, now what to do?

Intellectually, it is easy to see that the current living arrangement is not sustainable for much longer. But to actually consider what it will take to change these circumstances is painful. Think about the possible scenarios: spending time and money preparing the house for sale; figuring out how to downsize and dispose of many belongings; performing due diligence about where to move; assessing current health needs and trying to determine what the future might hold. Remember, these are just the first round of issues to address. Merely contemplating it is exhausting.

In her compelling book, *When the Time Comes*, Paula Span writes about a number of situations where adult children are involved in the care of aging parents. Paula points out that less than five percent of the elderly live in institutions of one type or another. Nursing home use has been falling for twenty years, even among those over eighty-five. Overwhelmingly, the people who care for seniors are the people who always have: their families.

Keep Span's comments in mind as you study alternatives. Better yet, obtain her book and study it carefully. Now, let's get methodical about the possible options that our hypothetical elderly couple may realistically consider.

## Stay Put

Why not just stay where you are? It's your home and you're comfortable there. Everything is familiar and none of that deadly downsizing is required. But, how do you do this?

Well, most cities have private registries, government agencies, home health care organizations, and private concierge services that can help with many of the chores elderly folks no longer want, or can, accomplish on their own. They can contract for everything from shopping, driving to appointments, assistance with daily chores, even walking the dog and undertaking home maintenance or repair services—if you have the financial resources. Some—perhaps most—will expect family members to provide the required in-home care.

Naturally, fees paid to non-family professionals vary greatly depending on the skills necessary to deliver the required services. Whatever the costs, they are in addition to those associated with living in the home.

Property taxes, utilities, and general household expenses will not likely decrease. The additional services obtained, from anyone other than family members, may prove to be quite expensive. A hard-nosed, realistic assessment of financial strength and cash flow is necessary before you choose this option.

While this alternative has the benefit of eliminating disruptive moves, selling the house and downsizing, there are some negative aspects, too. The only way to harvest equity in the home is likely to be a reverse mortgage, which may not fit in with overall financial planning and the current equity in your home. Should really extensive home health intervention be required, this option could get very pricey.

Finally, if skilled nursing or Alzheimer's care is eventually required, the home might not be a proper venue to administer that type of health service. Your health issues may force a move at a time when such a disruption is least convenient. "Staying put" may be a viable option, but it does carry many negative aspects. It should be noted that "people tell us again and again and again—they want to have the care they need brought to them in the setting of their choice. And the setting of their choice is not an institution," says Paula Span, quoting the AARP in *When the Time Comes*. In other words, "staying put" may be the first, and powerfully compelling, choice of many seniors in spite of possible impracticality.

**Move In with the Family**

This is probably a variant of staying put. Instead of remaining in your own home, you move in with a family member who can provide needed care. Paula Span cites the Urban Institute, which calculates that daughters and daughters-in-law provide an average ninety-eight hours of care a month, and sons and sons-in-law seventy-one hours to their aging parents. In *When the Time Comes*, Span states:

> Attempting to pay for the hours families voluntarily devote to eldercare, even at the low wages home health aides receive, would break the national treasury. AARP estimates the economic value of family care-giving in 2006, for disabled people of any age, at $350 billion, roughly equal to the total annual cost of Medicare.

Alternatively, the older person or couple may purchase a dwelling unit with the younger caregivers and both families occupy the home. Part of such a decision may be born of necessity; moving in with family may be the only alternative given financial circumstances and similar constraining issues. People do what they have to do, but it is painfully obvious that this arrangement can lead to a whole set of very difficult outcomes. Issues of privacy, conflicting lifestyles, and the effects on younger family members must be considered. Also, the possibility of never having respite from one another provides the opportunity to fray nerves and create serious conflicts.

While I am not dismissing this option, everyone must approach it with wide open eyes, saintly patience, unconditional love for one another, lots of tolerance, a flexible spirit, good humor, and a willingness to roll with the punches.

## Senior Independent Living Community

This is a broad category including "over fifty-five" housing complexes, clustered condominiums, or retirement communities. In most cases, moving to some sort of a senior community involves selling your home and occupying smaller quarters. Choosing this option is usually the beginning of downsizing from living independently in your own residence.

Beyond that, each type of community may, or may not, offer some amenities geared for a certain level of community life. For example, some retirement communities—homes, condominiums, or apartments—may provide common space for social interaction such as a separate great room or clubhouse. They may also be located near or adjacent to golf courses, tennis or swimming clubs, and other entertainment and leisure venues.

There may even be an activities director who arranges card games, potluck dinners, and trips to theatres, plays or other performances. These types of administrative services will often be billed as part of a monthly maintenance fee that also includes landscaping services for common areas, security, and other community activities found in most other condominium arrangements.

The obvious advantage of this alternative is that you have probably liberated the equity from your residence, gone through at least the initial step of downsizing, and begun the process of making new friends, most of whom will be of similar age to you.

You have still left yourself vulnerable to a sudden negative turn in your health, however. Most "over fifty-five" communities, of whatever organization type, do not include any provision for assisted living or any level of nursing service. If this need presents itself, you must still arrange for in-home service or, in more serious situations, seek a different place to live that does offer professional medical help of some kind. A second effect is living in a homogeneous environment made up strictly of older residents.

As with all other alternatives you will consider, moving to a senior community like this offers both advantages and disadvantages. In *When the Time Comes*, Paula Span provides a lengthy review of "intentional communities," which may be considered as a possible and innovative alternative to senior living communities.

## Assisted Living Facilities

It is important to define your terms when speaking about assisted living. The publication, *Choice: Resource Directory for Seniors in Oregon and S. W. Washington*, says,

> The term "assisted living" may be used to describe: (1) Personal and/or nursing services received in a retirement or assisted living community; (2) care received in an adult care facility or family home; (3) care received in certain areas of a skilled nursing facility; (4) care received in a private home.

Typically, these types of facilities provide assistance with many everyday activities such as dressing, grooming, bathing, toileting, eating and meals, transferring (getting in and out of chairs or beds), medication dispensing and monitoring, housekeeping, and laundry services. Obviously, choosing this alternative implies that you or your spouse is already debilitated at least to some degree, and not capable of total independent living. Again, we turn to Paula Span for her insight.

> Assisted living more often serves as a way station than a long-term home. Because seniors (often) wait until they're in their 80s, physically dependent, and cognitively impaired before they move in, they don't stay (in assisted living) long—just about 27 months, on average. The turnover is so high that of those celebrating at the Fourth of July barbecue, as many as 40 to 50 percent will not be there for the next Independence Day.

Span also talks about the quality she has observed in assisted living facilities: "I've encountered few people in the field who see the majority of assisted living residences as dangerous, or even of poor quality. They seem to be doing an okay job, overall. But it's an industry, one analyst told me, that 'overpromises.'" As the publication *Choice* says, a person needing this level of care may prefer a smaller setting such as an adult care home or small residential care facility.

\* \* \*

Each alternative offers positive and negative outcomes. There are certainly many options—like home sharing (mentioned above), adult care homes, skilled nursing facilities (when required), and other variations. Making final decisions about any alternative can create angst. You will find an excellent set of questions to ask yourself and the care providers when examining these options in *When the Time Comes*. You will also find there a wonderful set of information about resources related to eldercare. One thing is certain, however: Decisions forced on people by circumstance are less satisfactory than planned action.

Now, I want to tell you our personal story. I preface this with my clear bias. As I said before, my wife and I moved into Mary's Woods four years ago when we were in our early seventies. We went through the process of selling our home and doing the required downsizing. Since that time, we have had many conversations with friends and relatives who still live independently in their own homes and apartments. Frankly, a large portion of these people continue to think we were foolish to move. Their arguments come at us from many directions.

- "You two are both so young and healthy!"

- "Why would you want to live with a bunch of old people on canes, walkers and scooters?"

- "What did you do with all the lovely things you had in your home?"

- "You've given up your shop in the garage, your garden and so much freedom."

- "Gee—it costs so much money; how can you afford to live there?"

- "Aren't you giving up a lot of privacy?"

- "Where you live, death is just around every corner."

- "I don't want to interact with my neighbors every day."

- "I can count on my kids to help me out when that may be required."

- "You're going to cut yourself off from all your old friends and neighbors."

- "Eating institutional food everyday—I would hate that."

- And then the last, and most dismissive, comment always is: "Well, it might be a good idea for you; perhaps we will start to give it some thought in the next few years."

Here is a classic definition of old age: "Ten years older than you are today." Sometime between retirement and the onset of chronic illnesses that often occur in old age, most people develop a blind spot. They say to themselves: My spouse and I are getting along pretty well. Sure, we have some aches and pains but most people do in their late sixties or early seventies. We have planned our retirement income so that we can lead a comfortable lifestyle. We are still enjoying travel. Our home is comfortable and a perfect place to display all the wonderful things we have accumulated in our lives. We enjoy the freedom and opportunities for fun and relaxation that are presented to us in our lives. Yes, things are pretty good and *we expect them to stay that way for a while.* In other words, why should we change now, when things are going so well?

This is not only a false premise but a dangerous one, too. Time marches on inexorably. We may be drifting along on a tranquil river of life, but someplace ahead of us we are almost sure to encounter whitewater rapids or even a waterfall. No matter how much we may deny this fact, it is true that *nothing stays the same*. While we are healthy and vigorous today, it cannot stay that way forever. All of us know this intellectually, but we are reluctant to accept it emotionally. Acceptance of this truism forces us to face our mortality. It also forces a review of alternative future courses of action, some of which may be difficult or unpleasant.

I told you I speak with a bias. Since making our decision about our future—and we obviously believe we made the correct call—we have a two-part mantra that we earnestly impress on our friends: Make the move to retirement community living while you are still a couple. Do it while you are still able to deal with this major life change physically, emotionally, and mentally.

We can regale you with story after story about people who did not heed our mantra. Women have told us about trying to convince their husbands to move to a retirement community—with no success. Then, after the man died, the woman was forced to complete the move on her own. Believe me, it is a much tougher activity when doing it alone. Disregarding the second part of the mantra is even more evident. People wait, procrastinate, and dawdle until there is really no alternative left except leaving their homes and moving to a place that provides required care. We have many examples of folks who were absolutely overwhelmed just by the thought of organizing a move out of their home. Not only do they now lack the skills to plan such an event, but they cannot bear the thought of leaving their "stuff" and downsizing. In this case, the move often becomes a major problem for their children and grandchildren. There is seldom a satisfactory outcome when new living arrangements become a requirement instead of a choice.

* * *

Let's discuss the role children often play in this process. They sometimes have a blind spot, too. They may think of their parents as *getting older* but never *being old*. Then, one day, they look up and discover that their parents are old and frail. The children see that Mom and Dad are struggling with the daily chores of life, perhaps starting to have obvious memory problems and no longer able to handle all that is required to live in their home independently. This is both a sad and troubling moment for the kids.

The children begin the painful discussion about what to do. Finally, what I characterize as "The Telephone Call" takes place. The children get on a conference call together and attempt to answer the question: "What are we going to do with Mom and Dad? They can't possibly live by themselves in their house any longer." It may be too late to consider independent living in a retirement community. The physical and medical needs of the parent(s) may already be so great that a different level of care is required. A window of opportunity has been missed. Often this results in anxiety while the children move the parents from one facility to another as the care needs rapidly increase.

As I have reported, we have seen this happen in our own extended family. The kids may be required to expend inordinate amounts of time and effort trying to find new, appropriate care facilities as their parents' health quickly diminishes. This type of situation may create serious financial burdens, inordinate guilt, and a terrible sense of frustration as the children try to give their parents a reasonable and dignified quality of life in a downward-spiraling environment. In different circumstances, the children may recognize an impending need for their parents to get resituated while time and general health are still present. This is usually better than the first situation, but some parents may complain, "I'm living here in this retirement community because my kids forced me into it." This may still create problems, but ones which can be dealt with by everyone.

* * *

There is no denying that making a move into a retirement community—under the best of circumstances—is difficult and often traumatic. Most people will sell their home before moving in. That in itself can be a very difficult and trying proposition. What is the current state of the real estate market? Is the timing of the sale beneficial to the seller? Preparing the house for sale often requires "sprucing up," painting and executing long-deferred repairs. There is tension associated with keeping a house ready for inspection every day by potential buyers. Next are the final negotiations, which can be maddening and extended.

After the sale is completed, the action of getting all your goods out of the house is a major project. No matter how hard you work at it, there always seems to be one more closet, drawer, or cupboard to empty. All the while, you are trying to decide what to take with you to your new retirement home. Does this fit? Will I need that? Do my kids want any of my possessions? (Usually not.) What will I do with these heirloom pieces of china or crystal? You may be moving from a large home with three or four bedrooms, a living room, dining room, family room, kitchen, and garage to a unit with 800 square feet and one bedroom. You may conduct an estate or garage sale to help dispose of excess belongings. Getting ready for such sales is very hard work indeed. Finally, it is off in a borrowed truck to take the leftover stuff to Goodwill or St. Vincent de Paul.

The final escrow closing day arrives and you leave your empty house for the last time and move to your new retirement home. Don't forget—you're probably doing this in your seventies or eighties. The last several months of home-selling and preparation for the move have left you exhausted to the bone. And, as I said above, this scenario often represents the best of circumstances.

The next morning, you survey your new surroundings. There are boxes everywhere. You're confronted with the three phases of moving in: (1) physically getting all your stuff into the apartment; (2) finally getting all the boxes empty and things put away; (3) trying to remember what you brought with you and where you put it.

Nor do you know how to operate the thermostat to control the heat or cooling. You have to organize things like getting a phone system in place, figure out how to gain entrance to all the buildings and rooms with your key systems, finding out when meals are served, and where. Where do I get my mail? Who do I call if I need help with something? How am I ever expected to remember the names of all the new people I am meeting? In these circumstances, you would not be the first to feel a sense of panic, doom and utter discouragement. Hopefully, there will be some cheerful neighbors who will offer a hand, fill you in on all the "ins and outs" of the place and take you to dinner while introducing you to others who are also new.

I don't want to sound like Pollyanna but you *will* get through this rough patch. From observation, most new move-ins finally "come up for air" in about sixty to ninety days. No matter how tough things seem at the beginning, it does get better and you will begin to really enjoy your new home and surroundings. If you're like most, you will quickly conclude that moving to this retirement community was one of the best decisions you or your kids ever made. The people are generally very nice, the food is good, there are abundant activities (way more than you can participate in), you feel secure and safe, and you are in control of your own life. But the trauma associated with moving is not hypothetical; it is quite real.

❈   ❈   ❈

Many of the people I interviewed told me about their personal experiences in moving to Mary's Woods. As you will read, some of the stories weren't pretty.

Jeanne Wolf didn't have much of a problem with "stuff." But her move here from St. Louis forced her to leave four sets of friends from schools and activities that had been important to her. Jeanne also told me, "I hated to leave my doctors. Forming new relationships in a distant city was difficult."

Tye and Betty Lou Hutchens did have a little trouble with their stuff. "We had some books, antiques, and other sentimental items that were tough to part with," Betty Lou offered, "but like everyone else, we figured it out."

Cary and Lillian Coppock had a different problem. Cary said, "We had built our dream house on the water in Gig Harbor, Washington. We just *loved* our home; it was very hard to leave it." Lillian agreed: "We have never been hung up on stuff, but we do like to have nice things and this move meant we had to dispose of some of them. Like Cary, I adored our house and hated to leave it—but it has all worked out for the best."

Mary Bartholomew offered another perspective. "I had been in the same home for over fifty years. There wasn't a drawer, cupboard, or closet that wasn't jammed. Frankly, I was overwhelmed to even think about moving to a much smaller space. Fortunately, my children stepped up and figured out everything that needed to be done, what to keep and what to dispose of. I couldn't have done it on my own, believe me. Even my old neighbors came to visit and helped me hang the pictures that had come with me. Personally, my kids made my move stress-free. I am eternally grateful to them for their help."

❋   ❋   ❋

When speaking about moving from a home to some type of retirement housing, I have referred to "parents," "Mom and Dad," and "we" almost exclusively. This transition to retirement community living, however, is not just for couples.

As you have seen in the stories of my friends and neighbors, there are many single men and women who are enjoying healthy, vibrant and interesting lives. My focus is merely that my wife and I made this decision together and moved here with each other's help. Everything I am saying applies equally to singles. Soon it will be your turn to answer questions and objections from your friends who live "on the outside." Here is what you might say when you are faced with these questions.

*"Why do this when you're so young and healthy?"*

Yes, that's true and we are very grateful for that. But, you know, we might not stay healthy forever. We find it very comforting that our continuing care community allows us to utilize on-campus home health services or migrate from our current independent living status into assisted living, skilled nursing, and even a memory unit if and when we should require that in the future. We don't ever have to move again because of these medical and care options.

*"Why would you want to live with a bunch of old people on canes, walkers and scooters?"*

Well, we learned early on that our neighbors all had very interesting stories to tell and had led accomplished lives. Just about every new person we have met has enriched us with his or her life history.

We've also learned that each of us ages at a much different rate. We have met a lot of very young ninety-year-old people and a lot of very old folks who are seventy-five; you heard me say that before. A person is not defined by their cane, walker or scooter. Many are very talented, intellectually stimulating and a lot of fun to be with.

*"What did you do with all the lovely things you had in your home?"*

We sold them or gave them away. Our children really didn't want much of what we had except for small mementos. We thought a lot of the stuff was important, but learned that it wasn't.

We didn't want the final years of our lives to be focused on material things. We learned that hearses don't tow U-Haul trailers behind them. Our lives are not defined by what we have accumulated. We want our lives to be defined by who we are.

*"Haven't you given up your shop in the garage, your garden, and so much freedom?"*

That really isn't the case at all. We have a lovely, well-equipped shop on our campus. There are several people available to help me learn how to use the equipment and guide me through projects. I've actually learned how to do a lot more things since moving here.

As for gardens, planting areas are made available to those who enjoy growing things. It's fun to do your gardening in a relaxed social setting where your neighbor may be able to give you some tips that make your efforts even more successful. And, we actually feel freer since we no longer have worry about the care of our own home and property. The only problem we have encountered are the beautiful deer who roam our lovely campus—they are very fond of much of our produce and many of our flowers.

*"Gee—it costs so much money; how can you afford to live there?"*

When we sold our home, the equity we harvested was more than sufficient to cover the buy-in fee. In addition, most of the buy-in fee will be returned to our estate except in very unusual circumstances.

Planning for our move into this continuing care retirement community (CCRC), we carefully considered what would be covered by the monthly charges and what items would be eliminated as an expense to us. For example, we no longer have to pay property tax, a gardener, home repairs, utility bills (except for telephone), homeowner's insurance (replaced with a low-cost renter's policy), arborists, buying new appliances occasionally— the list of things we don't have to pay for is quite long.

On the other hand, lots of things are included in our monthly charges such as twenty meals per month per person in our dining rooms, maid service every two weeks to clean our apartment, a periodic deep-cleaning, all repairs and maintenance to our unit, a complete wellness center with up-to-date fitness equipment, a swimming pool, a long list of activities, medical and shopping transportation, classes, entertainment, exercise programs—that list goes on and on, too.

Finally, we received a substantial tax deduction since part of our buy-in fee and monthly fees are considered prepaid medical expenses and therefore deductible on our income tax. When we netted all the financial plusses and minuses after the first year in the CCRC, we determined that we had spent about $10,000 less on daily living items than we had the last year we were in our house. No, we don't think it is expensive to live here; it's a bargain. Sure, monthly fees will escalate about five percent per year, but that is comparable with normal inflation we all face.

*PLEASE NOTE: Every CRCC has a different financial model. You must examine the buy-in fees, monthly charges and what they cover, plus other financial considerations. It is up to you to determine the financial model at the different CCRCs being considered.*

*"Aren't you giving up a lot of privacy?"*

If you seek privacy (think Greta Garbo: "I want to be left alone,") it is very easy to find it here. All of us have a cocoon called our apartment or villa. You are not bothered by anyone in your own living unit. If you disdain the social interaction that occurs in the hallways, restaurants, wellness center, and other gathering places, that is your choice and no one will nag you about it. Early on in our stay, one veteran resident said to us jokingly, "You'll find that some of the inmates don't come out of their cells very often." All residents can certainly maintain privacy if they desire.

On the other hand, there are numerous opportunities every day to meet new people, swap life stories, enjoy one another's company over a shared meal and glass of wine and just celebrate life. As for us, the social interaction is one of the very best things about living in our retirement community. We have never felt so much a part of a vibrant community as we do in this place.

*"Where you live, isn't death is just around every corner?"*

For once, I agree with your premise. Yes, all of us here are old (whatever that means) and some are already quite infirm. Each of us has more years behind us than ahead. There are two ways of dealing with that reality. First, we can assume an attitude of impending doom and worry day and night about when the Grim Reaper is coming for us. That seems to me to be a pretty negative and gloomy way to anticipate the rest of our lives.

Or, we can awake each morning and count our blessings for another day, for time to accomplish some little—or big—objective, to enjoy our friends, to make a contribution to our world. To be death-denying seems pretty futile to me. All of us know, deep down, we won't get out of here alive. Why not savor each new day, hoping that our presence adds a small measure of happiness to someone else's life? Each of us has no idea when our last day will come. So why worry about it? Live life to the fullest as best you are able.

*"Don't you have to interact with your neighbors every day?"*

CCRCs are often described as "small communities where the streets are narrow and the houses close together." There is opportunity for daily contact with neighbors and friends—but privacy is also readily available.

This need for privacy is exercised in several ways. Some do not come to the dining rooms for meals. Others have no interest in participating in game nights or entertainment. Still others will take their exercise walking the grounds but do not come to the gym or swimming pool. Interaction with others may just not be their thing. However, that option is always your choice. While we would not opt for that approach, those who do find respect, not criticism.

*"Can't I just count on my kids to help me out when that may be required?"*

Of course you can; they love you and want what is best for you. But, is that what *you* want to do? Do you wish to burden them with caring for you while, at the same time, they are probably raising their own families and are at the most productive time in their careers? Do you want them to sacrifice a substantial amount of time (and, perhaps, money) diverting these resources away from their lives and focusing on you?

In some cases, that may be necessary, and often the children will step up and provide loving care for their aged, frail parents. After all, the parents might say, we took care of them until they were on their own. Why shouldn't they return the favor now that we need it?

Let's look at this a different way. When my wife and I decided to move into a CCRC, it was just before Christmas. We told each of our six children that our decision represented the most significant gift we had ever given to them. Never will they experience the gut-wrenching anxiety of trying to figure out what to do with us. We are in a safe place now. No matter what the future might bring we could receive the level of end-of-life care that we needed. The kids need never worry about that problem again. Some of our children had already gone through tough experiences with in-laws. They understood—and explained to their siblings—what a wonderful gift this truly was. Don't burden your children with your elderly care. They will be anxious and troubled enough as they walk with you to the end.

*"Don't you find that you are cut off from all your old friends and neighbors?"*

Come on, that's just nonsense. When you moved to a new home or town earlier in life, did you stop staying in touch with friends and neighbors? Of course, you may not see them as often, but you still maintain a relationship. Our CCRC is about ten miles from where we previously lived. We still see old neighbors and friends and delight in entertaining them here in our home and our community's restaurants. You will only be cut off from old friends and neighbors if you want to be.

*"Eating institutional food every day—don't you hate that?"*

We would tire of that, but we don't have to. We may be luckier than many, but our restaurants offer us a wide variety of well-prepared food served by young, attentive waiters and waitresses. Each night, in our main dining room, we have a choice of eight or nine entrees, several appetizers, salads and soups and luscious desserts. In the more casual restaurant, there is also a variety of interesting choices.

Recall I said that part of our monthly fee was twenty meals per person per month. Because we have a complete kitchen in our apartment, we often prepare several meals to eat at home during the month. We also take the opportunity to go to nearby restaurants for an occasional night on the town. Sometimes all of us hunger for good old comfort food—a tuna noodle casserole or spaghetti and meatballs. We make those at home and sometimes invite neighbors to join us in our unit for dinner. No need to eat institutional food every day if you are careful about choosing the right facility for your tastes.

*       *       *

We don't want to come across as self-righteous know-it-alls who have all the answers to elderly living arrangements. Frankly, it is easy to become preachy after you have lived in a CCRC for a while. We do sincerely believe that the last few years have been the best of our lives.

Everything is not perfect and we try to work with the management and staff to correct things that can cause problems. There is a residents' council and a number of committees of residents who are looking at every aspect of how we live our lives here. We don't run the place—a thoroughly competent board of directors has hired an excellent management staff to do that job. But, our voices are heard and often we can effect changes that we think are important.

We really care about our friends who are still living in their own homes. No, a CCRC is not for everyone. However, everyone needs to have a plan in place for dealing with advanced age. While the fact of aging cannot be denied, in reality, so many people are in denial about what might, could or will happen to them if they live long enough.

If you are considering "what's next," visit some CCRCs in your area. Ask questions. Have a meal there. Take your kids along so they can see the place, too. Get a rate card.

Attend one of their open houses. Observe the quality of community among residents and staff and how the two groups interact. Seriously think about how this type of arrangement might work for you. Good luck!

CHAPTER FOUR:

# DEALING WITH BODY, MIND, AND SPIRIT

*"Age is not a particularly interesting subject. Anyone can get old if you live long enough."*
—Groucho Marx

In a recent USA Today/ABC News poll of American attitudes about aging, the following issues represented the top three concerns facing those planning for the years ahead.

- Losing your health: 74 percent
- Losing the ability to take care of yourself: 70 percent
- Losing mental abilities: 69 percent

It is interesting that slightly more women than men are concerned about each of these issues. I'm not sure what that says about the men. The poll goes on to report the following general attitude:

> "Many Americans have this idea that as you age, your health will decline and you will not be able to care for yourself. Younger people fear old age because of a misconception that getting older means a rapid

decline in health," says researcher JaiMi Pennington of the New England Centenarian Study at Boston University. That's not necessarily so, he says. "More people today are living longer and healthier lives, and we can attribute that to advances in medical science and better nutrition."

My personal experience and those of my neighbors would indicate that Pennington's statement is mostly true. One striking example is my good friend Bob Rogers who, at age ninety, walks or hikes every day, takes no medicines as far as I know, plays very acceptable golf (and to his credit he defeats me regularly), is socially active, stays well-informed on current issues, still dabbles in his profession as a commercial real estate broker, is a lot of fun to be around—and has never been admitted to a hospital except as a kid for tonsils. What a role model he is for all the rest of us.

Of all my friends and neighbors at Mary's Woods, many seem to be fit, exercise regularly, eat healthful foods in appropriate amounts, and are careful to seek and follow professional medical advice. For the most part, the people I know are experiencing "active aging" with positive attitudes and trying to live each day allotted to them with grace. Statistically, at least, this probably adds up to a longer, healthier life.

Having said that, it is almost impossible for most of us to get into our late seventies, eighties, or nineties without being afflicted by some health issues. *American Fitness* magazine (September–October 1997) lists some of the physiological changes that may occur especially in sedentary adults that might lead to illness of some kind.

- Aerobic capacity decreases ten percent per decade.

- Pulmonary function decreases.

- Maximal cardiac output decreases.

- Muscular strength is reduced.

- There is substantial loss of muscle mass.

- Number of muscle fibers decreases ten percent per decade.

- Movement time and reaction time decreases.

- Bone mass decreases; body fat increases.

My understanding of others and myself tells me that, of all the age-related ailments, osteoarthritis is virtually universal. It's often painful, somewhat inconvenient—but, thankfully, rarely fatal. Almost all of us wear glasses because our eyes have diminished acuity. Some of us also deal with glaucoma or macular degeneration, which are more serious eye ailments. Hearing loss (there's a lot of denial about this) is rampant. My neighbors insist that hearing aides have a poor cost–benefit ratio; they are seldom reported to do very much good, even those that are outlandishly expensive. Many of us face elevated blood pressure and higher than normal cholesterol readings. Skin cancers—some mild, some more ominous—necessitate trips to the doctor and the telltale bandages on faces, arms and hands.

The single biggest problem, in my opinion, is the loss of balance and flexibility. Around here, falls are the number-one health concern. Everyone is worried about falling, so we often use canes, Nordic poles, and walkers to gain stability. It is also common to hear of hip and knee replacements, and the subsequent rehabilitation required. Cataract surgery is routine as well. Many people here are considered "bionic humanoids" because they are so full of replacement parts.

Most of the local pharmacies deliver prescription drugs ordered by Mary's Woods residents. It's quite a sight at the end of the day—shopping bags full of medicines awaiting pickup at the front desk by the residents; abundant pills, salves, and drops to alleviate, stabilize, or cure a host of ailments. We are clearly a highly medicated population. My observations are strictly non-medical judgments; I'm sure our doctors would be much more competent reporters of our health status.

Of course, what I have mentioned here are mostly generic health issues. Most people do their best to shrug off as many difficulties as possible. I guess we think that's what "aging gracefully" is all about. When meeting others in hallways and common areas, it is the standard to greet people with, "How are you?" or, "What's new with you?" The typical response is, "I'm doing great," or, "Everything's super!" Now, both parties know that this exchange is merely polite and friendly. While many people honestly think of themselves as "fine" even in the face of illness or handicap, both also understand that they probably share a lot of aches and pains, but this is rarely discussed in general conversation.

One day in a hallway, a neighbor said to me, "You know, we should really say 'I love you' when we meet in the halls. At our ages, what are the chances that we might not see that same person again?" A provocative idea. I don't consider the thought morbid or dark; he is merely trying to say that we are all in this aging business together and should therefore treat one another with great love and gentleness.

* * *

David Snowdon, PhD, in his fascinating book *Aging with Grace*, comments that many people still believe that, as we age, our bodies and minds wear out. This is a myth, says Snowdon. The book *Aging with Grace* is often referred to as "The Nuns' Study." Snowdon extensively tracked the lives of several hundred women belonging to an order of Catholic nuns called the School Sisters of Notre Dame. His work produced significant data especially related to the overall health of those women who lived similar lives. The book provides fascinating insights about the substantially different health profiles of these nuns as they aged.

John Donne was right: "No man is an island, entire of itself." When someone begins the long, slow fade into Alzheimer's, for example, the ripple affect touches many others. We have about thirty people in our special memory unit called Caritas House. All of them are experiencing the scourge of dementia—some in earlier stages and others very advanced. It is quite painful to watch someone visit their spouse in Caritas, to speak with them, to help with feeding or just to be present. Recently, three men whose wives were in this unit began meeting weekly for dinner. Each of them was experiencing their own personal anguish; sharing these personal difficulties with one another probably made the situation a little easier. But, more importantly, seeing the three men eating together was a great inspiration to the rest of us. The other residents referred to these men as "The Three Saints." They provided a wonderful example, because those of us observing all recognize the possibility that one day we, too, could face something similar either as caregiver or the one being cared for. We live in hope that this does not happen to us.

Many folks are facing serious health concerns like Parkinson's disease, cancer, multiple sclerosis, stroke, diabetes, various forms of heart disease, depression, shingles and, perhaps the worst of all, some form of dementia including Alzheimer's disease. Of course, I haven't listed all the ailments we face, but you get the picture. In almost every instance, the afflicted individual is only one of many people affected by these diseases. The spouse, the children and grandchildren, friends, and neighbors and the staff all feel some pain along with the person who is ill.

*     *     *

Regarding the onset of a disease, we often hear the question "Why me? What did I do to deserve being afflicted with _____ (you fill in the blank)." Again, I must stress that my observations are not supported by medical knowledge; I am just reporting what I and other residents have seen. Through general reading, interaction with our own doctors and readily available information, we know that many diseases are often familial, that is, passed from one generation to another in our genes. For example, my father died of prostate cancer. I contracted it, too. Therefore, according to all reliable literature, my three sons possess better than a 90 percent chance of having prostate cancer in their lifetimes. Many similar things can be said about other inherited diseases.

Then there are those which seem to strike randomly, and when we least expect them. After the shock of hearing the diagnosis in the doctor's office, we begin to wonder what we could have done to prevent it—if anything. While none of us can be totally immune to all illness—we all must die of something—there are probably some things we can do to live longer, healthier lives. I offer nothing really new here; we all know the prescriptions to follow even if we sometimes fail to do the things we know we should.

*Diet*

A lifelong regimen of eating a modest amount of food seems to do wonders for longevity. Being thin is good; being obese is not. The calories we consume should be dominated by fruits, vegetables, whole grains and items low in saturated fats. Fish, skinless chicken and legumes are better for us than red meat. Natural foods are healthier than processed things. Salt and sugar should be used in moderation. We already know this; unfortunately, some of us don't follow the plan as we should. Why?

Because a rare sirloin steak and a baked potato covered with sour cream and butter followed by a crème brûlée may be more appealing to our taste buds than a small piece of broiled fish, brown rice, and broccoli.

As we know, our human nature often leads us off the track. There is little doubt, however, that the discipline of a healthy diet will make a substantial contribution to our chances for a longer, healthier life.

A word about alcohol consumption. Many of today's elderly grew up in a time when a drink was socially acceptable and a common occurrence. And those who are widowed may experience loneliness and turn to alcohol more than they should. Yet, it is possible for things to get out of hand quickly, and lives at all stages have been ruined by excessive drink. Among my friends and neighbors, most enjoy a glass of wine with dinner and perhaps an occasional mixed drink in their apartment before coming to the dining room. While the great majority do not over-drink (at least, I don't see a problem) there is still potential for serious difficulties with alcohol. It is important to remember that we do not metabolize alcohol efficiently in our older age. Where a drink or two in our forties or fifties might have posed no problem, the same quantity of alcohol might pose all kinds of dangers now. This is not a temperance lecture, however; this is merely a word to the wise. If you are over seventy you should understand that drink of any kind will affect you more now than when you were younger.

David Snowdon in *Aging with Grace* makes an interesting and provocative statement that asks us to expand our view of eating.

> What I know for sure is that nutrition for healthy aging is not just about eating certain foods or downing a certain number of milligrams of a prescribed number of vitamins each day. It also depends on

where we eat, whom we eat with, and whether the meal nourishes our heart, mind, and soul as well as our body.

So, we must address not only the type of food and drink we consume. We must also consider the setting in which it is taken, who joined us for the meal, what we discussed, the laughs we shared, the insights exchanged. The shared meal is central to lives well lived.

I was forced to address my own weight issue recently. My annual physical indicated that my blood glucose level was creeping up; without intervention, the doctor told me I was on the way to Type II diabetes. I consulted a diabetes nutritionist and followed her suggestions carefully. Reducing serving sizes, cutting way back on carbohydrates and similar things helped me to reduce my weight by twenty-five pounds very quickly. This resulted in normal blood readings and much lower blood pressure and cholesterol readings. I was also able to continue on to lop off another thirteen pounds.

*Exercise*

David Snowdon in his book *Aging with Grace* says, "Wherever my speaking schedule takes me, someone in the audience nearly always asks, 'What is the most important thing I should do to age successfully?' 'Walk,' I reply."

We often hear reports advising that regular daily exercise of thirty minutes or more may lead to a dramatic reduction in the onset of many diseases including heart conditions, diabetes, cancer and other sickness. But, let's face it: exercise can be tedious, boring, uncomfortable, sweaty, hard work and generally not much fun. Most of us have little trouble finding an excuse to avoid exercising. "I'll do it tomorrow," we tell ourselves. Tomorrow comes and we usually find yet another excuse.

In our well-equipped wellness center at Mary's Woods I am often struck by how few of the residents utilize the facility. I'm sure many satisfy their exercise needs by walking around our beautiful campus. However, winter has its share of inclement weather, when walking is neither safe nor comfortable.

I personally believe the biggest obstacle to exercise is a failure to make it just another part of our daily routine. We sleep; we eat three times a day; we bathe and groom; we use the toilet; we set aside time for reading, amusements, interaction with others—why not schedule our exercise, too? Exercise is best completed at about the same time each day so that it conveniently fits your daily schedule.

Exercise is especially important for those of advancing age. We have more porous bones, our balance is not what it once was, and our joints are often creaky. Nothing can help alleviate these conditions more than regular exercise. As important, exercise assists in keeping our aerobic function and metabolism high. This, in turn, helps us to fight off the extra pounds that often creep up on us in our later years. Exercise is close to a miracle cure for many things that can negatively affect our health. A final benefit: Exercise helps our self-image. Healthy bodies are very important. Healthy minds and serene spirits are equally important to our overall well-being.

*Intellectual Stimulation*

At the beginning of this chapter, I quoted from a USA Today/ABC News poll stating that many people were worried about losing their mental abilities. It is a common belief that, as we age, our mental abilities diminish. I'm not talking about dementia or Alzheimer's—most think that even healthy old timers don't process mentally as well as they used to. While this may be true anecdotally ("Grandma can't remember the birthdates of all fourteen grandchildren anymore,"), who cares? There are many studies showing that proactive older people can keep their gray matter healthy and active.

Dr. Rob Winningham of Western Oregon University spoke to a group a Mary's Woods residents about the work he was doing with elderly brain function. His research suggests that brain matter and the synapses that connect parts of the brain can actually be restored in the elderly. He pointed out that activities like learning a foreign language, doing crossword or Sudoku puzzles, working with computers, playing complex card games like bridge, engaging in art classes, and similar behaviors could improve brain function.

We have so many residents at Mary's Woods who are interested and involved in these types of activities. We are often provided with opportunities to attend lectures or concerts, get involved in various types of artistic projects like painting, sculpting, book making, visiting cultural sites and participation in writers' workshops, among other things. There are many avid readers who share books and make extensive use of our library. It is remarkable how vibrant, alive and "with it" most of our population is. Do these people ever forget a name, miss an appointment or draw a blank as they walk down the hall with no idea where they're headed or why? Of course! But, we know lots of thirty-somethings who do the same things.

That is not to say we sometimes observe, with profound sadness, a beloved neighbor or friend who begins to show the symptoms of dementia. While we hate to see this happen, we do take comfort in knowing that there is a caring place in our facility that will treat them with loving tenderness when that need arises.

### Lifting Our Spirits

What of our spirits? We often hear about the negative aspects of getting older. What are the positives? SeniorResource.com lists a number of ways that our spirit may be enhanced when we reach elderly status. Included are the following:

- Creativity that we learned earlier in life does not diminish with age. If we were good artists, sculptors, or writers when young, we will be even more so with aging.

- Normally our ability to cope increases and our stress levels decrease. We have pretty much seen it all and most of us can "roll with the punches" better when we are old.

- We learn to take more responsibility for our health. We have figured out what to eat and how much exercise we need, and we act on that knowledge with prodding from others.

- We understand ourselves better—we are comfortable in our own skin—and seem to have a better perspective on life and events. We may be more patient with others.

- We are more confident about ourselves and care less what other people may think of our opinions and actions. This helps us not get our feelings hurt quite so easily.

- We know better what it takes to satisfy our own wants and needs. We aren't so uptight about "keeping up with the Joneses."

- Our capacity to love increases as does our curiosity and altruism. Along with this, our levels of anxiety diminish.

- Gratitude deepens. We become very thankful for all life's blessings that have been—and continue to be—poured out on us.

- We may be more relaxed sexually.

- Often, our sense of humor is heightened.

All the people I spoke to while preparing this book had some fond memories of their earlier years. There were many joys associated with beginning a career, starting a family in some cases, and gaining additional professional competence. I asked them to also tell me about newfound joys experienced in these last ten to fifteen years.

Dorothy Gornick, a family friend who lives in Sheldon, Washington, was quick to answer: "I have made so many wonderful new friends in the past few years. They are terrifically important to me." Dorothy resides in a manufactured home park. At age ninety-eight she is almost totally blind but still lives independently. While she relies on friends to help her out, she is more of a giver than a taker.

Virginia Campbell has derived great pleasure from being a part of the Mary's Woods family and the new relationships that has created. "So many things give me joy," Virginia said. "I love to do Origami, write limericks, observe my grandchildren and great-grandchildren grow and expand with their educational opportunities."

Lillian Coppock told me, "My greatest joy is that my children all married Christians and they are raising their families the way we raised them." Cary Coppock chimed in, "My greatest joy is being with Lillian for all these years."

Philip Martin found post-retirement joy in training other ministers in interim ministry skills for helping congregations make the transition from one pastor's style to that of another. Philip told me, "It helped to reorient their changing community and our changing cultural context." I also asked about newfound losses, but I will save those responses for a later chapter.

Pablo Picasso once said, "It takes a long time to become young." And that is one thing we might strive for—to be young in our old age, at least young in spirit. In *Facing Age, Finding Answers*, Ardis Stevenson writes that we should not fear getting old. We should ignore the common notion that only young people are carefree, and life in old age becomes less and less satisfying. I certainly agree with this premise; being positive about the status of our age is a good thing. Stevenson concludes, "What's the point of being a grouchy ninety-year-old pessimist anyway?"

I was fascinated with the answers given to me when I asked our residents, "Are you optimistic about the future?" Hilda Kullberg, comfortably seated in her favorite chair surrounded by her own lovely watercolors and paintings said, "Yes, I am optimistic about the future, especially my own. I have a very positive medical profile, seem to eat moderately and keep moving."

Jeanne Wolf had an opposite view. "I'm worried about the direction being taken in our country," she said. "What are we leaving for our children and grandchildren?" Jeanne's animated comments and flashing eyes indicated her sincere concern. "I also worry about the ability of children to concentrate. The whole world seems to be made up of thirty-second sound bites."

Edith Pattillo, a lovely, reserved and well-informed resident was anxious to point out to me the beautiful landscape paintings her spouse had created while he was alive. Her apartment, located on the ground floor overlooking a peaceful apple tree orchard provided a serene outlook. Edith mirrored the feelings of Betty Lou Hutchens. Both women professed a general spirit of optimism but were quick to agree that long term health issues can dampen their enthusiasm. Betty Lou's spouse, Tye, agreed: "I try to stay optimistic but memory loss and other health issues sometimes make it difficult."

Dorothy Martin offered an interesting metaphor: "I'm optimistic but don't expect things to always go smoothly. You know, winds activate an element within trees that makes them grow stronger. I believe the 'winds' people face gives those folks the opportunity to build their strength."

Another aspect of our spirit is our spiritual life. I am not speaking about organized religiosity, although adherence to denominational creeds along with frequent community worship is important to many devout people. There are also some here who may be agnostic or atheist; even those beliefs may be considered as statements about their spiritual life or lack of one. No value judgments will—or should—be made about anyone's religious beliefs or non-belief. I wish to speak to the underlying *spiritual* nature of most human beings.

Transcending our denominational practices, most of us have some deep-seated spiritual underpinnings. Over the years, through contemplation, prayer or observation, we have attempted to answer some of the great fundamental questions of life: What is our purpose here on Earth? Is there a supreme being? What is my relationship to this primal spirit? Do I believe in life after human existence? If I do believe in an afterlife, what do I expect it will be like? Do I possess a soul as well as a body? What obligations do I owe, if any, to all the other human beings on earth? Do I fear death?

Since my neighbors and I have lived longer than we are going to live, I wanted to explore their views about the greatest event of life—death. Again, some of my neighbors offered heartfelt thoughts about the meaning of religion, spirituality, and death to their own lives. For example, Sister Kathleen told me, "I have no fear of death but, of course, I wonder how I will do when I come right up against it." Yes, how will we react when we realize we are living our final earthly days or hours?

Steve Korsak hesitated for some time before giving his response. "I do worry about a long death process. Like everyone, I would like to avoid pain. From a human viewpoint, I will miss my friends and loved ones."

On a lighter note, Steve said he wouldn't mind being like a specific famous person. "The Queen Mother of England was born into royalty, lived to be 103, and died in her sleep. How can I get a ticket like that?"

Lillian Coppock exuded great confidence in the afterlife. "Do I fear death? Absolutely not! I have great faith in the Lord." Lillian is a deacon in her church and often visits those who are near death. "Almost always," she said, "life ends peacefully. God cares for us."

Sterling Dorman was equally positive. "I don't fear death, even the circumstances. Of course, I'm not sure anyone can ever be completely ready."

Reverend Philip Martin told me, "If my life ended today, I would think of it as just another transition to face." With a slight grin, Philip also noted that many people may feel ambivalent about death, like Woody Allen, who was reported to have said, "I'm not afraid to die but I don't want to be there when it happens!"

Famous philosophers and spiritual leaders have filled the world's libraries with answers to the great questions about life and death and other equally profound concepts.

As part of our aging health profile, our spiritual side needs to be serene. Each of us may find this serenity in diverse places using different means. Organized religion is but one way people find the peace they seek. We may also ask ourselves: are we reconciled with everyone who has passed through our life? Are there any agendas I need to complete before my life on Earth comes to an end? Is there any anguish, fear, or doubt that I need to overcome before my time is up? We cannot see or touch this aspect of our aging, but our spiritual dimension is every bit as real as our flesh and blood.

*     *     *

Many of us may be uncomfortable thinking or speaking openly about end of life issues, about our eventual death. Henri Nouwen, in his magnificent book *Our Greatest Gift: A Meditation on Dying and Caring*, writes,

> Is death something so terrible and absurd that we are better off not thinking or talking about it? Is death such an undesirable part of our existence that we are better off acting as if it were not real? Is death such an absolute end of our thoughts and actions that we simply cannot face it? Or is it possible to befriend our dying gradually and live open to it, trusting that we have nothing to fear? Is it possible to prepare for our death with the same attentiveness that our parents had in preparing for our birth? Can we wait for our death as for a friend who wants to welcome us home?

Yes, as we age we must be concerned about our physical, mental, and spiritual lives. Each plays a most significant role in who we really are. There is no way to describe a human being with a mere statement of physical form and shape. Every facet of our *being* must be included to adequately state who we have become. Whether tall or short, thin or portly, handsome or not-so-much—that is just a part of the story. To completely describe someone requires that we discover a range of virtues, weaknesses, traits, charisms, fears, hopes and dreams. We look to find courage, persistence, patience, joy, kindness, compassion, empathy. Only when we have discovered the *whole person* can we say: ah, yes, I know him; I know her. This is an important part of the autumn phase of our lives. We first must get to know ourselves; once completed, this may allow us to get to know others. If this happens, we now have met someone we can walk beside to our final destination on the road of life. Remember our mantra: We're all in this together.

.

# CHAPTER 5:

# **SOME FINANCIAL CONSIDERATIONS**

*"Nobody knows the age of the human race but everybody agrees that it is old enough to know better."*

—ANONYMOUS

Like it or not, your personal financial situation directly affects which retirement alternatives are open to you. I wrote early in this book about my own epiphany occurring at age fifty. I was cruising on the economic superhighway, earning good money and supporting a large family. But I was not providing enough for an adequate financial retirement plan for my wife and me. This type of planning is very personal; indeed, each person or couple will have unique requirements.

The crucial element to *every* plan is that it must be started early enough to have a chance of being executed successfully. Realize that we eventually reach an age where we are no longer able to catch up with our previous failure to save money for retirement. To avoid this problem, replace haphazard direction and fuzzy thinking like, "We have got to start saving and investing more!" with well-thought-out goals and objectives containing precise timelines and unfailing adherence to the plan's specific action items.

The biggest problem for many people is that they are unsure how to get started. If you fall into that category, excellent help is available—and most of it is free. Lists of retirement planning websites are available on all Internet search engines. Three popped up in my research for this book as especially clear and comprehensive: Union Plus Retirement Planning Center (retirement.unionplus.org), the Retirement Planning Calculator at www.retirement-income.net, and the Financial Planning Toolkit (finance.toolkit.com). These sites—and many others—will guide you through what you must consider and accomplish to get a retirement plan in place. They also provide the calculators necessary to do the math that will underpin your plan.

*      *      *

Below is a summary on developing a retirement plan. While I believe the precise financial aspects of a plan are most important, there are other non-financial considerations that affect the financial ones. Answering the following questions will lead to more detailed analysis of your situation.

*What is your vision of retirement?*

What are the kinds of things you want to accomplish in your retirement years? Can you articulate any lifelong goals that you want to achieve? What do you look forward to in retirement? What do you feel will be the least satisfying part of retirement?

*Where do you want to live?*

Is staying in your present home an important objective? Can your home be adapted to meet health challenges you may face in the future? Are you interested in moving to another city or state? What are the things that would attract you to this new place? Are you looking forward to travel in your retirement? Where do you want to go? Do you have friends or family to travel with?

*Whom do you want to spend time with?*

How do you plan to meet new people? How important to you are things like time spent with family, friends, educational pursuits, hobbies, sports like golf or tennis, travel, or working part time? Do you find volunteering fulfilling?

*How long to you want to continue working?*

Would you be interested in starting a new business? Have you calculated how much money you might need in retirement? Have you estimated how much money you will have in retirement? Do you feel comfortable that you have done sufficient planning for retirement so far? What is your greatest concern when considering retirement?

* * *

These are the general questions to get you underway with your plan. Discuss them thoroughly with your spouse and make sure you two are in agreement on the major issues.

We have many neighbors here who are widows. Some have told stories about how they tried to talk their spouses into coming to a retirement community—in most cases, without success. The husbands were reluctant to give up their shops, gardens, and the perceived freedom of living independently in their own homes. Then, fatal illness or sudden death followed, leaving the widow to make the move on her own. Most of the women are not bitter about this; it is more a sense of wistfulness about what might have been. Many know how happy their spouses would have been living here and they regret that they did not get to spend at least some contented time here with their spouse. Yet their situation does highlight the need for starting early on a retirement plan and reaching consensus before fates overcome the events of life.

All of this planning hinges on your age when you begin in earnest to execute your financial retirement plan. As the laws of compound interest clearly indicate, the younger you start, the better off you will be at retirement age. But we also know how hard it is to save and invest when you are younger. I have always advised my children that it was smart to save ten percent of their gross income; if they did that from age twenty-two, they would probably have a million dollars by the time they were sixty, even if they did not have especially high-paying jobs or were not particularly aggressive investors. There are hundreds of savings calculators available on the Internet. They make it easy for you to figure out how much you must save on a consistent basis in order to reach a specific financial goal.

No matter at what age you begin your plan there are a number of elements to consider. Again, you may find quite opposite views of how a plan should be constructed. Let me discuss some of the things I think you must address to structure a comprehensive financial retirement plan.

*Household Budget*

Without being obsessive-compulsive, you need to have a good idea about where and how much income you are generating and how that money is being spent each month. Don't go crazy accounting for every pack of gum or cup of coffee; conversely, keep track of general categories of expenses fairly closely, such as housing-related, food, entertainment, transportation, utilities and telephone, taxes, medical, charitable contributions, and general expenses like petty cash, work-related items, and other similar things.

If you go nuts recording every nickel you will soon become discouraged and give up your budget—and that is a problem. Consider some of the simple home computer accounting programs that are available. An hour or two a month with your pay stubs and checkbook can provide some sophisticated reports that will show you how you are doing.

*Emergency Savings Account*

Everyone needs to have some money tucked away to weather unforeseen adverse events. Temporary layoffs at work, sudden medical expenses, auto repair costs after an accident, storm damage to your residence that may require extensive refurbishing—things do happen "out of the blue" and you must be prepared to deal with them.

How much should you have in this fund? You will hear widely differing views, but I believe this savings account should total between three to six times your gross monthly income. With these funds in hand, sudden events may deal you a body blow, but you may be able to roll with most punches.

## General Savings and Investments

Here's the part that will test your mettle. Especially with younger people, you may be just starting your family, raising children and trying to provide for their education, buying a home, acquiring the material things you consider important for a pleasant lifestyle—all the while trying to climb a corporate ladder, rise in your profession, or operate a business. In this stage of life it often seems that, no matter how much your income may be, you just can't seem to save money and keep up with your bills, too. I am going to suggest a mantra for you to ingrain in your personality:

*Gross Income – Planned Savings = What I Can Spend*

Most of us get that exactly backwards. We figure that *gross income minus our expenses equals what we can save.* I think that is wrong and will, if followed, often lead to disappointing savings or no savings at all. From our youth, we have all heard the idea "pay yourself first." That is what my mantra suggests you do. If your philosophy is only to save what is left over, you won't save much. There is always relentless pressure to spend more, buy something else and—oops! There is nothing left over for our savings account. "Oh, well," we say, "I'll catch up on my savings account next month." Sure you will!

Here's the point: What you save, invest and compound prior to your retirement is likely to be a significant share of your total retirement financial resources. With the ongoing public debate about the financial integrity of Social Security, Medicare, Medicaid, and other tax-supported entitlement programs, no rational person is going to count on the government to support them entirely in their old age. You are going to have to do a lot of the heavy lifting yourself.

*How Much Money Will I Need?*

This number is a moving target. I again note that you will find many different plans on the Internet; you should choose to follow those that feel comfortable to you.

I will make one specific observation: Many plans will advise you that you will need less money in retirement than you did beforehand. I don't necessarily agree with that advice. Yes, a case can be made that certain expenses, pre-retirement, will diminish or disappear after you have left the workaday world. On the other hand, you may wish to do some things—travel, education, hobbies—that will consume more financial resources. In addition, as you age it is possible that medical expenses may increase. Personally, I think you need to plan on having resources that will provide you with 100–120 percent of your pre-retirement income. But the answer to this vexing question is not so clear cut as a simple percentage.

In my book, *Common Problems; Common Sense Solutions*, which is directed to the owners of small and mid-sized businesses, I discussed the issue of "defining financial security." Here is what I said:

Several years ago, there was a somewhat amusing but extremely poignant essay in the New York Times Sunday Magazine section. The essay examined the issues related to "The Number"—defined as that amount of money when invested at conservative rates of return that would support your definition of a "life of leisure." The fundamental premise of the essay was that "The Number" differed for most people. For example, someone that had worked hard all their life in a modest job might say, "Gee, I could retire and live a life of leisure, by my standards, if I had $50,000 of annual income." To someone in that circumstance, having $50,000 coming in every year—without work—might allow them to experience a wonderful retirement filled with pleasures only dreamed about during a work-a-day life. Assuming that a 5% after tax return was a conservative rate of return, we calculate that a nest egg of $1,000,000 would provide the desired $50,000 of annual income. (For this discussion, we will assume that the principal amount is never invaded or reduced). To someone else who experienced more prosperous circumstances during their working life, "The Number" might be substantially higher. Again, for example, a person who worked in a high profile executive position providing significant income might say, "To continue my lifestyle and do some of the other things I've always dreamed about will require $250,000 in annual income. This will permit me to give generously to my church and university and enjoy first class travel to parts of the world I have not seen." Using our same investment criteria, "The Number" for this individual would be $5,000,000. You can see from these two simple examples that "The Number" would have infinite variations depending on the wants, needs and desires of any person. Here is the real question: What is "The Number" for you and your family? Investment advisors constantly suggest to us that we understand what our future needs will be.

Much of what I wrote in *Common Problems; Common Sense Solutions* is relevant to a financial retirement plan—but not all. You do not have to create "The Number" entirely on your own. Part of the answer to "how much money will I need" will be provided by Social Security, pensions (perhaps), defined benefit plans like 401(k)s, IRAs, annuities and other sources. When planning for how much you need, don't forget to factor in a provision for inflation. Keep in mind that a generally modest inflation factor of three to four percent per year will virtually double your need for money over a twenty-five-year period.

*Social Security Benefits*

You need to know how much you will receive from Social Security when you retire. The Social Security Administration has a helpful website that will show you how to figure out what benefits you will receive, when you can begin receiving them, and how they may be taxed. I again point out that what is current information today may change in the future because the financial integrity of the system is threatened by many factors. But, you must start somewhere, so determine what your projected benefits might be. How you factor in contingency plans may be tricky.

*Employee Pensions*

You may be the beneficiary of a company or government pension. Check with the personnel department where you work to determine how much your pension will be, when you can begin collecting, what vesting conditions exist, what portion of the pension is guaranteed, and whether the pension is indexed in any way for inflation. Get all the relevant information you can so you might include this information in your plan.

## IRAs and Defined Contribution Plans

Your employer may have provided an opportunity for you to open an IRA or Defined Benefit Plan like a 401(k). If you are a small business owner, you may have established a Simplified Employee Plan (SEP). These funds may permit you to accumulate retirement funds on a tax-free basis (check with a tax advisor to confirm this).

It is important that you understand how these plans will work for you at retirement, how you access the funds, and what are the IRS requirements about the timing and amount of withdrawals. If you are fortunate to have this type of investment vehicle, it will assist in your financial resource planning for retirement. If you are able to contribute tax-free to any of these devices, it is probably wise to make the maximum yearly contribution permitted by law.

## Annuities

An annuity is the only other financial instrument, besides a pension, that can provide a guaranteed income in retirement. There are two types of annuities: fixed and variable. Fixed annuities pay their buyers a guaranteed stream of income at a fixed rate. Variable annuities are insurance-based investment contracts that grow tax-deferred until you begin taking withdrawals from them. Variable annuities are sensitive to stock market trends and, therefore, are somewhat volatile.

*The Wall Street Journal* produced a comprehensive Guide to Annuities on November 11, 2009. It is worthwhile reading. Importantly, the article asks and answers ten important questions related to buying an annuity. Find out if this is a viable investment for you.

*Home Ownership*

Most people who have lived beyond forty know that the residential real estate market is cyclical and volatile. It is comforting to think that the value of a home will always increase, but the debacle of 2008–2009 reminds us that this is not the case.

Home ownership is the bedrock of our American Dream, and over the long term can become a good investment— especially if you acquired it on conventional terms that did not leave you overly leveraged, and with monthly payments you can comfortably afford. While I will stipulate that timing of the sale can make a huge difference in the proceeds, your home can be an important contributor to your final retirement resources. If you have a home, keep an eye on comparable sales in your neighborhood. This will give you the very best idea of how much yours may be worth.

Assuming you do have a home, it can become a significant financial resource when you reach retirement. Absent unusual circumstances, you will not have children living with you at that time. You may have paid off your mortgage or at least see the end of payments in sight. Even if you plan to stay in your home, a reverse mortgage may be appropriate if you wish to harvest equity from the property. In our case, the sale of our home provided the buy-in fee at Mary's Woods with money to spare.

*Estate Planning and End of Life Documents*

I shake my head in disbelief when I discover someone at or near my age who has failed to take care of end-of-life matters in advance. It goes without saying that everyone should make the time to engage legal counsel for the preparation of wills, trusts (where appropriate), powers of attorney, health care directives, and other associated documents. And, yet, so many fail to take care of this basic task.

I can report many sad stories of financial chaos that besets families, especially widows, when someone dies suddenly without the proper legal documents in place. Don't wait until you're "old" to handle this. Young parents should complete this work as soon as the children arrive— at the latest. Updates to a thorough plan can be made along the way.

Please don't put this task off, no matter your current age. In addition, it is so helpful to a surviving spouse and family if lists of service providers like attorneys, CPAs, and insurance agents are available along with such things as the location of bank accounts, investment advisors, insurance policies and even final funeral requests. It is not morbid to do this; it is practical. It also is an important piece of your retirement planning documents.

＊　＊　＊

These nine topics are like a retirement plan recipe. You must assemble the ingredients and mix them together carefully, in a way that creates a program you understand and are comfortable with. This combination may require some outside advice. As I have mentioned, there is quite a bit of that counsel available to you via the Internet. The final objective is to create a plan that shows you how you can live the autumn phase of your life with some degree of comfort and peace—and, hopefully, not outlive your money.

The residents at Mary's Woods were quick to share their feelings about the issue of money.

Almost all whom I interviewed said virtually the same thing: they were worried about outliving their financial resources and the implications of that possibility. With varying levels of concern, Ish, Wilton, Vic, Hilda and Jeanne all felt they had been prudent and conscientious about financial planning. The realities of general inflation and the dramatic increases in healthcare costs were quite worrisome. Jeanne Wolf commented that some residents were in denial and "had their heads in the sand" about finances.

Other residents stated: "We have tried to plan very carefully and *think* everything will work out OK—but you never know, especially when you attempt to forecast future health care needs or our national economy."

Mary Bartholomew was more upbeat: "I can live within my income. I don't worry about this part of my life." Others also reported that did not feel any unease about their financial situations.

No matter how well one plans, it seems that dealing with financial issues can be troublesome. I also should mention the question of financial scams involving senior citizens.

The July 2009 edition of *Northwest Senior & Boomer News* discussed the many ways scammers try to take advantage of seniors. These crooks will try anything to part the elderly from their money, including promising to qualify them for federal stimulus funds, re-financing mortgages, bogus "work at home" job offers, home improvement schemes, and debt relief through credit counseling, among many others. What can you do, as a senior citizen, to protect yourself from these unscrupulous characters?

- Make sure you ask your bank about procedures to protect your credit cards in the event of theft, loss, or misuse.

- Close accounts that may have been tampered with.

- Make sure businesses supply you with information about all transactions charged to your account.

- Frequently check your credit reports with the three major credit bureaus.

- Place your credit reports on a "fraud alert," which alerts you to new applications for credit requested in your name.

The absolute bottom line about scams is to never give out personal information, social security numbers, or credit card numbers to anyone you don't know, either in person or over the telephone.

Finally, there is the issue of long term care insurance. The purpose is to provide a source of funds to pay for home health care, assisted living and other types of custodial care, which can become very expensive.

I am not an insurance expert; you must seek the advice of a professional to determine what, if any, coverage might be appropriate for your circumstances. However, there are a few overall concepts I am comfortable sharing with you. First, it is obviously much less expensive to arrange for this insurance when you are younger. There is a negative component to acquiring this insurance early on—your policy coverage may become obsolete by the time you need it. Still, most experts would tell you that earlier is better than later.

Second, make sure you are buying policies from financially stable, highly rated insurance companies. Company ratings are easily obtained from Standard & Poors, A. M. Best and Moody's. Features of the policies that you may wish to look for in any policy include:

- The daily benefit paid is in line with the costs for custodial care in your state or region.

- There is some kind of an inflation rider.

- There should be at least four years of coverage; the typical stay in assisted living is approximately two and a half years.

- There should be broad coverage that includes assisted living, home health care, or custodial care.

- The policy should be guaranteed renewable for life.

- The plan should be "qualified," that is, premiums paid are tax-deductible.

\* \* \*

What I have presented is a "tops of the trees" review of the major things to consider in creating your course of action. Even with prudent and careful marshalling of resources, savings can be eaten away by relentless inflation. In addition, many of us are living longer lives thanks to medical science and our own adoption of healthy living protocols.

There are few greater sources of stress than realizing that next year, your expenses will exceed your ability to pay. This chapter, therefore, is an urgent call to the reader to get serious about his or her own financial plan for a future living in retirement. It is unfortunate that one must spend so much time and energy thinking about money, but this is a practical reality. The single, most important message of this chapter is don't delay, do not wait, to create a specific financial retirement plan. It will not take care of itself.

CHAPTER 6:

# PETALS ON A FLOWER

*"Old age is defined as doing more and more things for the last time and fewer and fewer things for the first time."*
—ANONYMOUS

Evie and I attended a seminar on aging several years ago. The presenter said memorably, "Whatever you were when you are younger, you will be the same in your old age—except more so." Since many of our parishes' lay ministries involved visiting the frail, elderly, and homebound, we got firsthand corroboration of this truism.

Another concept from the seminar stuck with us, too: We heard that old age is like a beautiful flower—vibrant, colorful but also somewhat fragile. When we become old, we suffer a series of losses. These losses are like pulling petals off the lovely flower one by one.

Dear friends die. Remove a petal. Then we lose beloved siblings. Remove another petal. Our driving privilege is revoked. Our spouse is taken from us. We no longer hear well. Our sight deteriorates through macular degeneration or glaucoma. Our health restricts our travel—something that was once the highlight of our lives. Remove a whole group of petals. Nights are frequently very long because sleep is difficult. Arthritis leaves us with chronic pain, hands that no longer work well, and misshapen feet. Hips and knees need to be replaced and rehabilitation is long and arduous. Every three months we trudge to the dermatologist who finds skin cancers during each visit, some ominous. We contract Parkinson's disease. Heart arrhythmias suddenly appear. Memory seems to abandon us frequently. We bear with the inconvenience and embarrassment of incontinence. Cancer strikes. There are torn rotator cuffs. Falls are common and often dangerous. Tasks that were easy just a few years ago are now a chore. Fatigue is daily. Multi-tasking is a thing of the past. Everything takes longer than it used to. Remove the remaining petals.

Our beautiful flower is no longer quite so lovely. It seems that a seniors' major social life involves making and keeping doctors' appointments and attending funerals or memorial services. Friends and neighbors confirm that they are experiencing losses, too. While I spoke to them, these perceived losses tumbled out of their conversation emotionally, staccato like. Sometimes old age can provide a toughness that shields us from hurt or loss. But it was obvious to me that my neighbors needed to share this part of their lives with me, however small the slice.

June McAllister said it was tough losing a daughter-in-law to ALS (Lou Gehrig's disease). "There must be a reason for this, but it's hard to know," said June.

Steve Korsak told me, "I miss myself! Parkinson's takes a real toll."

Another resident said, "I miss time the most."

Hilda Kullberg stated, "I yearn to be playing golf and not being tethered to canes and walkers."

"It's a loss for me not being able to attend the opera anymore but the auditorium does not have railings on the steps, so I can't navigate," offered Jeanne Wolf.

Bob Henry said, "It was a terrible loss when my nineteen-year-old grandson died."

Betty Lou Hutchens has had both her sisters die. "A crushing loss," she called it.

"Not being able to just 'get up and go' is a loss for me," reported Lillian Coppock.

Sister Kathleen told me, "First, I lost my mother and then two of my brothers. Finally, when I had cancer, it was a terrible shock—it certainly changed me!"

And these are called the Golden Years? Is there any good news here? Please!

I don't want you to think that everything about being a senior citizen is a negative "downer." Old age—and old people—are not single beautiful flowers; each person is a complete bouquet filled with beautiful textures, vivid colors and life-affirming characteristics. This is not some altruistic mush; I see these gorgeous bouquets every day I live here at Mary's Woods, in my witnessing the lives of other residents. By and large, old people are upbeat, happy, interested in others and full of good cheer. They tend to be patient with their neighbors, possess a good sense of humor, and are eager to find ways to make a positive contribution to the community. They enjoy good food, love an occasional sip of wine to go with it, laugh at stories they have heard frequently, and happily tell everyone about their grandchildren. On a lovely summer's day they walk around the beautiful campus, observing God's magnificent creation at every turn. They look forward to their exercise program three days a week. After dinner they can be found playing cribbage, pinochle, bridge, Scrabble, and poker.

The art room is usually filled with people doing watercolors, sculpting something or creating other works of art. The woodshop is full of people doing leaded glass, re-caning chairs, or repairing furniture for another resident. Musicians practice together on their instruments. A theatre troupe practices for their next performance. The Marie Rose care center has many visitors—residents looking after their neighbors, who have just returned from surgery for rehab. The Monday evening wine social and sing-along is always crowded. Many gather around the piano to sing familiar old songs from their youth—"Sweet Rosie O'Grady," the "Whiffenpoof Song," or "Someone's in the Kitchen with Dinah." It is often sung badly but nobody cares; everyone is too busy having fun.

The wine glasses are filled at the bar. ("Up to the rim—I may not have a chance to get back for a second glass.") The dining room doors finally open and the diners file in for a delicious dinner and more conversation and stories about life, former travel adventures, grandchildren—and a little innocent conversation about Mrs. Green down the hall; and isn't it interesting that she and Mr. Jones seem to be having dinner together quite frequently. What a delicious little scandal that could turn out to be! Most re-tell stories told many times before, but that's OK since their dinner partners can't remember all the details, anyway. When the dessert tray arrives you often hear, "I know I shouldn't but that Boston cream pie looks awfully good tonight; please bring me a piece."

Dinner over, everyone stops by the mailroom to see if there is anything in their federal or internal mailboxes. Most folks broadcast the daily complaints: "All the mail I get is junk stuff. Why don't the kids ever write anymore?" They do, but it is in the form of an e-mail. Grandma or Grandpa would prefer a stamped envelope to a computer file. And then it's off to sign up for the next tour or class, or to play card games, or to attend the evening entertainment or visit the library. There's always something to do— enough so that one often forgets about that arthritis pain or worry about the grandchild's education or the upcoming medical appointment with the oncologist. Maybe it's off to the apartment to watch "Jeopardy" or the "Lehrer Report" before switching to more reading on the current book. Bedtime arrives after the late evening TV news, hopefully accompanied by sleep.

One way or another, the hours pass until the sun peeks over the Eastern horizon and a new day has arrived. Some may greet the dawn with a little prayer: "Thanks for giving me another opportunity at life. Help me to be productive and use this time wisely and generously in service to other members of this community."

Yes, a new day has begun. Like the ones before—and those to come—this day will be full of activities, pleasures and friendship with some challenges added to the mix. At day's end there will be a full measure of contentment and happiness for most residents.

Does this general chronicle sound like a group of old

people wallowing in the miseries of aging? I can only report what I know and see. Yes, my view may not be thoroughly representative of what aging is about for everyone. A community like ours often looks like a bell curve. Naturally, there may be a few extreme characters at both ends, but the majority falls into the middle ground; they are just normal, good-hearted, accomplished, and interesting folks. Like any community, you are attracted to some people more than others, but isn't this true of most groups? What I want to convey is that the autumn phase of life can—and should—be full of meaning, joy, happiness, productivity, humor, and love of neighbor. Does that only occur in a community like Mary's Woods? Of course not, but it is what I observe here daily.

While never denying that life is terminal, I see people doing their best to make every day a consequential event. Everyone knows that some of their neighbors or friends may be experiencing certain anguish—physical, emotional, psychological, or spiritual. Along the way, those difficult times visit us all. Every day brings triumphs and tragedies, smiles or tears, to someone in the community. Today may not be your turn, but it will surely come to you, because that's the way life is. Empathy can be seen everywhere, and people help each other with the little tasks of life. Today I may be the giver; tomorrow I must receive—and believe me, it is much easier to help than to be helped.

* * *

In spite of a general mood characterized by a chin-up, shoulders-back, let's-be-positive view of life, you can sense a patina of melancholy in the community, too. Friends whose eyes sparkled with life and enthusiasm for years slowly, almost imperceptibly, begin to dull and take on a vacant, not quite focused look. Previously productive, energetic, interesting, and fun—lives slowly diminish before our own eyes. It is terrible to see a once lively friend experience this slow but obvious decline. Pinched faces tell of chronic pain; slightly imprecise speech and a labored search for words indicate that brain function may be slipping. Admissions to hospitals and our skilled nursing unit become more frequent and closer together. Are we headed towards life that is less independent and more reliant on others? But isn't that why we came here in the first place?

Yes, we came to this place because we envisioned a seamless path from independent living to assisted living and, finally, to higher levels of care as our needs changed. Intellectually, it is very comforting to know that this progression—if it is needed—comes with a minimum of disruption, since all care levels are offered within the same facility. But, in practice, many may not wish to make the move from independent to assisted living.

Why? Because, as Paula Span writes in *The New Old Age* blog in the *New York Times*, "To leave an independent living apartment means not only losing one's home and social network but also part of one's identity... there is a certain level of stigma involved...there are social boundaries." In other words, the transition from independent to assisted living may not be as seamless— or effortless—as we originally thought. Span further notes that promoting interaction between independent and assisted living residents may not work, either. For example, "Independent living residents don't like [sharing a dining room]. They view themselves as healthy and active. They want to feel like they're in a nice restaurant conversing with friends; they don't want to be faced with those in declining health."

I have seen some evidence of this at Mary's Woods. There has been not-so-quiet grousing about "all the walkers and mobilized chairs in the restaurants." I also know of some independent residents who vigorously oppose moving from their cherished apartment homes. Would they hide illness or physical difficulty from friends, neighbors, and staff to avoid this move? I'm not sure. While we embrace the concept of continuing care, the practical reality is that it may not be as easy or painless as we thought to move from one place to another. As Paula Span says at the conclusion of her blog entry: "Having to leave home is disruptive and distressing, it seems, whether you are moving seven minutes or seventy miles away."

I must admit there are some negative aspects to living in a community like ours. I hate it when final indignities, especially the loss of independence, affect my special friends. I just *hate* it. There is also a sense of helplessness in certain situations—there is absolutely nothing I can do to assuage someone's physical or emotional pain.

I have a close friend whose spouse is deteriorating quickly. He is deeply disturbed to see her in such a difficult situation and shares her pain, at least emotionally. In addition, he himself is facing serious health issues. How I would love to help him! Other than being present to him, there is *nothing* I can do.

CHAPTER 6: PETALS ON A FLOWER

Another dear friend recently died. His wife is distraught. Evie and I try to show her our care and concern, but we don't seem to be effective in helping soothe her grief and loss. When these situations arise, it seems that death or disability may be more imminent for us all, and I selfishly say, "I do not want to lose my friend! I don't want them to suffer in any way!" And yet, as Henri Nouwen says in *Our Greatest Gift*:

> Nothing makes all human beings so similar to each other as their mortality. Tragically, however, we think about death first as an event that separates us from others. It is departing. It is leaving others behind. It is the ending of precious relationships, the beginning of loneliness. Indeed, for us, death is primarily a separation and, worse, an irreversible separation.

Instead of seeing just the negative, it is important to also grasp the positive. Evie has taught me a very important lesson. When I become depressed over the loss of some friend, she has reminded me, "Don't forget, you would never have met these wonderful people if you hadn't moved here. Just think of all the joy and pleasure their company provided while they were in good shape and available."

* * *

So many living here as my neighbors have such an uplifted and positive view of life. I queried them about what kind of legacy they think they will leave. More specifically, I asked what might friends and family say about them when it is time for their own funeral or memorial service? Essentially what I was asking them to do was to write their own obituaries. The answers were intriguing—but often invoked long pauses.

"I hope people will remember me as loving and compassionate," said Sister Kathleen. "I have tried to maintain friendships with diverse people who are often marginalized by society. I would like that to be recognized."

One person told me, "I want people to say I wasn't boring."

Bob Henry was very clear about his legacy. "It is my family. Family reunions were the high point of my life. I have been so pleased to see the kids and grandkids get along so well."

Edith Pattillo hopes someone remembers that she loved bridge. She would also be pleased if someone said, "She was a force for good and I enjoyed her company."

Dorothy Gornick said she hoped people might say, "She always tried to see the other's point of view and helped people think about all their blessings."

Margaret Dillon guessed that there would be three things said of her: "She never stopped talking; she was a survivor; she thoroughly enjoyed life."

When I posed this question to Virginia Campbell, an icon at Mary's Woods because of her vibrant life at age ninety-nine, she paused and looked around her apartment, her gaze resting briefly on the many works of art in the room completed by she and her children. She then focused on me with her piercing, brown eyes. In a soft but firm tone Virginia said, "I hope they remember that I spent my life as a civic volunteer. In the last few decades, Herald and I spent tremendous amounts of our time, energy, and even our resources to make our community better for all its residents. Isn't that what life is supposed to be about? If that is how I am remembered, I would be pleased." Her serious expression was quickly replaced with a soft smile. "Just let everybody know; I plan to be around for a while longer yet."

Once again, I turn to Joan Chittister's book, *The Gift of Years.*

> What we are inclined to forget is that each of us leaves a legacy, whether we mean to, whether we want to or not. Our legacies are the quality of the lives we leave behind. What we have been will be stamped on the hearts of those who survive us for years to come. What are we leaving behind? That is the question that marks the timbre of a lifetime.

Those of us who have reached "senior" status have faced good times and bad during our lifespan. I was interested to know about the biggest challenge that my neighbors had faced in the last fifteen to twenty years. Steve Korsak said, "Of course, my Parkinson's has been a major 'hit.' But, not all the effects are negative. I have learned to be more relaxed and willing to listen to others' point of view. I think the disease has made me more humble and helped me into a period of self-discovery."

Vic Christiansen stated that his seriously handicapped son "created a terrific challenge for my wife and me." Vic also said, "My own physical deterioration has been tough for me to deal with."

Bob Henry sadly reported, "What could possibly have been a greater challenge for me than seeing my dear wife, Jean, slowly die of Alzheimer's? That was extremely stressful."

Tye and Betty Lou Hutchens were in agreement: "Trying to maintain good—at least adequate—health is a major challenge. Both of us would dread being invalids."

Echoing Bob Henry's statement, Dorothy Gornick said her greatest life test was "dealing with my husband Tony's Alzheimer's disease."

Sterling Dorman told me her challenge related to a close relative. "My sister-in-law was severely mentally handicapped. She required a lot of care and it was a situation we could not control—but it did control us."

Margaret Dillon was emotional when telling me of her life's greatest test—trying to maintain a healthy relationship with her in-laws. "It was terribly stressful. I was very hurt by their actions."

One interviewee said her stress related to leadership forced upon her. "I am essentially a shy person but was often called upon to lead, especially related to fundraising efforts. This was very hard on me."

Think about the stressors in your own life. They can sap your energy and leave you wilted. Personally, I find it difficult to ignore my own personal stress. How am I doing with my own health issues? Am I being an attentive, understanding spouse and companion to Evie? Are my children doing okay in their careers and family relationships? Are our grandchildren learning good moral values? Will our financial resources support us to the end of our lives? Some stress issues can be managed; others are beyond our control. So, I live with this attitude: Yesterday has come and gone—nothing I can do about that now; tomorrow is not here yet so why worry about it? Live in the present—it's all I have. I'm not sure this avoids stress but it assists me in having a positive perspective. Each of us should do what we can to avoid or manage stress in our lives.

＊　＊　＊

Right or wrong, the aged are considered by many to be wise. So I also asked my neighbors if they were willing to offer any advice to those approaching retirement age. I asked, "How would you advise these folks to lead their lives? What specific things would you recommend that they do?"

Margaret Dillon was short and sweet: "Keep the faith; get all the education that you can; never pay rent."

Mary Bartholomew suggested, "Practice voluntary simplicity; live below your means; save for retirement, but don't forget to share some of your resources with the less fortunate."

One woman offered: "Live each day as well as you can with the most energy you can muster and don't forget to develop some hobbies and outside interests."

Dorothy Martin urges, "Keep all relationships 'cleaned up' as you move along. Every important contact with family needs to end with 'I love you.'"

Sterling Dorman advises, "Look forward to new, exciting opportunities; find time to do volunteer work; share whatever you have with those less fortunate; welcome new friends and ideas into your life; travel when you can; enjoy your family."

Tye and Betty Lou Hutchens said, "Do your best to save three times as much as you think you will need in retirement."

Virginia Campbell said, "I should know—don't let vanity get in the way. Use walkers and canes to get around; accept what life brings."

Jeanne Wolf had simple advice: "Guard your integrity; be kind; protect your health."

Hilda Kullberg said, "Do some good in your life and don't be selfish, especially to the less fortunate."

Vic Christiansen wants us to "slow down, be thankful for the moment; volunteer if you can. Couples, remember there is no 'you,' only 'we' or 'us.'"

Wilton Jackson offered some practical advice: "Buy an extended care health insurance package when you're younger and the premiums are lower."

Steve Korsak advised younger people to "be less serious about life; don't try to be in control—because you're not!"

Ish Murray proclaimed: "Don't be too quick to give advice or try to tell people what they should do."

Finally, my personal suggestion. Remember, everyone you meet is superior to you in some way. Do your best to learn from every single person you encounter throughout your life.

*     *     *

In our old age we often make deep and abiding friendships with those in our community of aging people. We delight in their company, their stories, their good humor, their apparent and remarkable gifts shared with all they encounter. If these friends are taken from me, I think, I shall be devastated by the loss of pleasures and good times I shared with them. But, as Henri Nouwen says, we are all in this thing together. If some friends leave me first, I will desperately miss them. My time for leaving will come soon enough. I must not think of these losses as final endings, devastating separations, or tragic conclusions. In proper context, these departed friends were most esteemed because of their gracious personalities, amusing stories, unique achievements, and the unconditional friendship they extended to me and others. I will miss their human presence; I celebrate and honor their lives well lived full of success, courage, integrity, and tender care for their families, friends, and loved ones.

This should not be a time of loneliness or separation but a time of happy remembrance for those wonderful people who so enriched my life but now rest in peace. I must focus on the fact that they lived their allotted span of days the best they could. To a portion of that time, I was a witness. Finally, I again turn to Henri Nouwen's *Our Greatest Gift* for inspiring words:

> What a gift it is to know deeply that we are all brothers and sisters in one human family and that, different as our cultures, languages, religions, lifestyles, or work may be, we are all mortal beings called to surrender our lives into the hands of a loving God.

So, there it is. We examined the continuum of human life from conception, birth, childhood through young adulthood, heading on through middle age, to old age, and finally the death that ends our physical life on earth. As we proceed through life, each phase offers new experiences and challenges. This book has been about navigating through the final phase of life in a graceful, courageous, and even inspirational way.

How can we sum up what the autumn phase of life is all about? It is a time when we move from self-reliance to more dependence on others. It is a time of newfound joys, but also difficult losses. It is a time when we can solidify our legacy for future generations. It is a time for community, for love of neighbor, for sharing our talents with others. It is a time for giving of ourselves, especially caring for those who need our gentle attention. It is a time for courage in the face of physical and mental diminishment. It is a time to spread good cheer and humor to our family, friends and neighbors. It is a time to ask big questions about the purpose and meaning of life, to seek intellectual satisfaction about an afterlife (if we conclude there is one), and to ponder our specific reason for being on Earth at this time and place. In short, we get to be the star performer in the final act of a unique play—one that displays our life's journey with its highs and lows, euphoria and depression, laughter and tears, triumphs and tragedies. May God bless us all and guide our steps on this challenging, complex, and wondrous journey.

# AFTERWORD

I was fourteen years old when my dad and mom agonized over "placing" (that was the word they used) my grandfather in a nursing home. Walt was a gentle soul who had loved deeply, smiled freely, and believed in living life to its fullest. My parents had second thoughts about this move, but Granddad insisted—and eventually they all agreed that a nursing home was the wisest choice.

I was surprised and saddened at my first visit to his new home; he had lost that mischievous twinkle in his eyes and his contagious smile was reduced to a forced grin. I remembered thinking, "Doesn't anyone understand that Granddad won't thrive on just bingo?"

Seventeen years later, Grandmother Maggie accepted the same fate. With a heavy heart she moved into a retirement home and, like Granddad, quickly lost her spirit for living. Life became merely an existence and was far from thrilling for her.

Only a few years ago, my mother-in-law, Lois, suffered an unexpected, temporary health scare. Together, Lois and I began exploring living options for an independent senior. We discovered a continuing care retirement community (CCRC) in her area that was clearly the best value. It provided the most vibrant atmosphere and long-term comfort. I was impressed especially with the CCRC's holistic lifestyle, which focused on nurturing the mind, body, and spirit. Lois liked the idea of community living with a continuum of care. Even though the CCRC was totally dissimilar to the nursing homes she had visited long ago, she couldn't shake the long-term emotional association with those "traditional" settings.

Furthermore, Lois was afraid to leave her home. "Giving up your home," she argued, "means giving up your freedom." She finally chose to remain in hers. It was a decision she gradually learned to regret as she faced the growing burden of home ownership and increasing isolation from friends and social activities right up to her death. I so wish she had been educated earlier in her life about CCRC living. She would have flourished—socially, emotionally, and physically—in such a community.

I am deeply grateful to Greg Hadley for this book. Not only does he provide sound advice, but he has advanced the efforts of educating our senior population and their families about the advantages of living in a continuing care retirement community.

May we celebrate age and celebrate life!

*Cheri Mussotto-Conyers*
Director of Marketing
Mary's Woods at Marylhurst

# SELECTED BIBLIOGRAPHY

Bernard, Jan Selliken R.N. and Miriam Schneider, R.N. 1996. *The True Work of Dying.* New York: Avon Books.

Collins, Kelsey. 2008. *Exit Strategy: Leaving this Life with Grace and Gratitude.* Sisters, Oregon: ChaseHawk Publishing.

Chittister, Joan. 2008. *The Gift of Years: Growing Older Gracefully.* New York: Blue Bridge.

Hadley, Greg. 2004. *Common Problems: Common Sense Solutions.* iUniverse Publishing.

LaFarge, John S. J. 1962. *Reflections on Growing Old.* Fort Collins, Colorado: Roger A. McCaffrey Publishing.

Lewis, C. S. 2005. *Made in Heaven: And Why on Earth it Matters.* New York: HarperCollins.

Nouwen, Henri J. M. and Walter J. Gaffney. 1976. *Aging: The Fulfillment of Life.* New York: Doubleday.

Nouwen, Henri J. M. 1981. *Making All Things New.* San Francisco: Harper & Row.

Nouwen, Henri J. M. 1994. *Our Greatest Gift: A Meditation of Dying and Caring.* New York: HarperCollins.

Nuland, Sherwin. 1993. *How We Die: Reflections on Life's Final Chapter.* New York: Vintage Books.

Skinner, B. F and M. E. Vaughan. 1983. *Enjoy Old Age.* New York: W. W. Norton and Company.

Snowdon, David, Ph.D: 2001. *Aging with Grace.* New York: Bantam Books.

Span, Paula. 2009. *When the Time Comes.* New York: Springboard Press.

Stevenson, Ardis. 2008. *Facing Age, Finding Answers.* Trafford Publishing.

# ADDITIONAL RESOURCES

*Selected Websites*
This is a small selection of Internet sites providing retirement calculators, information about financial planning, and guides for selecting senior living arrangements.

www.fidelity.com
www.retirement.unionplus.org
www.finance.yahoo.com/retirement
www.retirement-income.net/retirement-plan
www.articles.moneycentral.msn.com
www.online.wsj.com/public/page/news-retirement-planning
www.seniorcitizenhousing.net
www.aplaceformom.com
www.seniorresource.com

*Selected Articles*
Following are some publications and specific articles that were part of the overall research material for this book.

*Choice, Resource Directories for Seniors in Oregon and S. W. Washington*, 2008–2009.

Finnemore, Barry. July 2009. *Northwest Senior & Boomer News.* "How Scammers Take Advantage of You."

Greene, Kelly. 2009. "How to Navigate Medicare If You're 65 and Working." *Wall Street Journal*, July 11.

Kelly, Tom. 2009. "Seniors on the Move Have a Lot of Factors They Need to Consider." The Oregonian, July 12.

Market Watch from Dow Jones, *Retirement Weekly*.

McClanahan, Larry. July 2009. *Northwest Senior & Boomer News*. "Are You Strangling the Goose That Lays the Golden Eggs?"

Myers, Randy. 2009. "Will You Have Enough? A Guide to Annuities." *Wall Street Journal*, November 11.

Pflug, Jack. July 2009. *Northwest Senior & Boomer News*. "Help Available For Those Unsure About Medicare Benefits and Limitations."

APPENDIX:

# **INTERVIEW QUESTIONS**

1. Was there a specific time when you said to yourself, "I've gotten old?" When did that happen? Were there special circumstances?

2. What is the most significant change—physical, emotional, psychological, attitudinal or spiritual—you have noted in yourself in the past ten to fifteen years?

3. If there were one thing you could do over in life, what would it be?

4. Have there been any newfound joys for you in the past ten to fifteen years? How has this changed your perception about life? Also, tell me about the most significant losses you have experienced during the same time period?

5. Are you currently hopeful and optimistic about the future? About your health? About your financial future? Why or why not?

6. Given all the alternatives available, why did you decide to move to a place like Mary's Woods? Was there one overriding reason for your decision? How much did your family influence the decision?

7.  What was the greatest stress caused by the move? Was there a single most difficult thing for you when moving from your home to Mary's Woods? Was your "stuff" an issue for you?

8.  Now that you are in the twilight of your life, do you have any fears as you squarely face your mortality?

9.  What one or two specific pieces of advice would you give to someone in their fifties or sixties facing their own retirement?

10. Are you generally satisfied with what you have been able to accomplish in your life and the legacy you will leave?

11. What has been life's toughest challenge for you, especially in the past fifteen to twenty years?

12. Have you ever experienced a major epiphany, the "ah-ha" moment that forever changed the direction of your life? What was it? When did it happen to you?

13. Other than a spouse, has any one person been extremely influential in your life? Why, or in what way?

# ABOUT THE AUTHOR

Greg Hadley with his wife, Evelyn, lives in Mary's Woods at Marylhurst, a continuing care retirement community located in Lake Oswego, Oregon.

After completing his undergraduate education at the University of San Francisco, finishing his MBA studies at Pepperdine University, and attending the Harvard Business School, Greg spent his professional life in the business world. He worked for IBM and was General Manager of Computer Sciences of Australia. Then, for twenty years, Hadley and his partners were involved in acquiring, operating, and selling industrial companies. After moving from California to Oregon in 1990, Greg established a thriving management consulting practice, spent time as a college educator, author, and a professional public speaker. Now retired from his business interests, Greg is still involved in civic, political, and community volunteer activities.

Greg spent thirty-nine years as an amateur baseball umpire, mostly at the NCAA Division 1 level. He is the author of four previous books. *Fundamentals of Baseball Umpiring* (Perfection Form Company, 1981) is displayed in the National Baseball Hall of Fame, Cooperstown, New

York. His second, *Common Problems; Common Sense Solutions* (iUniverse, 2004) is directed to the operators of small and mid-sized companies. The third, *100 Everyday Epiphanies* (Wine Press Publications, 2005) is an acclaimed prayer book. Finally, *God's Words to My Heart* (BookSurge, 2009) is a devotional book based on sacred scripture. For further information or details, please e-mail greg@gbhadley.com.

Made in the USA
Charleston, SC
21 April 2010